Thomas Moe, DMin

Pastoral Care in Pregnancy Loss: A Ministry Long Needed

*Pre-publication
REVIEWS,
COMMENTARIES,
EVALUATIONS . . .*

"**T**homas Moe's treatment of this misunderstood but frequent need among our families is a critical contribution to the pastoral care literature. He comes at the issue with more in-depth understanding than most, having experienced this kind of loss in his own family, and having interviewed a significant number of parents who have suffered either miscarriage, stillbirth, or neonatal loss. He estimates that only 75 percent of all conceptions result in successful live births, so the frequency of this type of loss far exceeds what one might expect.

Moe believes strongly that ecclesiastical communities can do a much better job as caregivers to this kind of need. We too often misunderstand, minimize, and neglect this kind of loss. Thus, many parents are harmed by our attitudes, and left drifting from one church community to another without adequate response to their pain and grief.

The various coping styles of parents are addressed, and Moe includes a helpful section on the incongruency between one parent's grief and another's, a condition that drives them apart."

Dr. Nils C. Fribert, PhD
Professor of Pastoral Care,
Bethel Theological Seminary,
St. Paul, MN

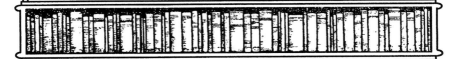

"**A**s a registered nurse caring for bereaved parents, I have learned of parents' disappointment in the support they receive from their pastor and parish. *Pastoral Care in Pregnancy Loss* provides excellent information not only for the pastor but for parishioners as well. Pregnancy loss resources for pastors are minimal. This book is a wonderful addition to the RTS Bereavement Services resource list and bibliography when doing our RTS counselor training courses for clergy and other professionals. I appreciated the author's handling of spiritual questions regarding the death of a baby through miscarriage, stillbirth, or newborn death. Spiritual issues are concerns of health care providers, and this book can help anyone have a better understanding of the dilemma bereaved parents face when their baby dies before or shortly after birth."

Bonnie K. Gensch, RN
RTS Bereavement Services Coordinator,
Gundersen Lutheran Medical Center,
La Crosse, WI

"**S**urprisingly, society, seminaries, and many clergy have much room to grow in their care for bereaved families whose babies die in pregnancy loss. *Pastoral Care in Pregnancy Loss* is a welcome and needed resource to aid spiritual counselors in their understanding and growth in this long-ignored arena.

The book builds a clear and powerful case for why families grieve after the loss of their baby and explores what coping resources they may need. It offers gentle yet forthright suggestions on how to counsel these families. As a mother who has suffered such a tragedy, and as a support person for thousands, I wish this book were required reading for every pastor. If this care were more widely modeled in our communities, the healing that could occur would be tremendous."

Sherokee Ilse
Author, *Empty Arms* and
*Giving Care, Taking Care:
Support for the Helpers*

The Haworth Pastoral Press
An Imprint of The Haworth Press, Inc.

Pastoral Care
in Pregnancy Loss
A Ministry Long Needed

THE HAWORTH PRESS
New, Recent, and Forthcoming Titles
of Related Interest

Growing Up: Pastoral Nurture for the Later Years by Thomas B. Robb

Religion and the Family: When God Helps by Laurel Arthur Burton

Victims of Dementia: Services, Support, and Care by Wm. Michael Clemmer

Horrific Traumata: A Pastoral Response to the Post-Traumatic Stress Disorder by N. Duncan Sinclair

Aging and God: Spiritual Pathways to Mental Health in Midlife and Later Years by Harold G. Koenig

Counseling for Spiritually Empowered Wholeness: A Hope-Centered Approach by Howard Clinebell

Shame: A Faith Perspective by Robert H. Albers

Dealing with Depression: Five Pastoral Interventions by Richard Dayringer

Righteous Religion: Unmasking the Illusions of Fundamentalism and Authoritarian Catholicism by Kathleen Ritter and Craig O'Neill

Theological Context for Pastoral Caregiving: Word in Deed by Howard Stone

Pastoral Care in Pregnancy Loss: A Ministry Long Needed by Thomas Moe

A Gospel for the Mature Years: Finding Fulfillment by Knowing and Using Your Gifts by Harold Koenig, Tracy Lamar, and Betty Lamar

Is Religion Good for Your Health?: Balm of Gilead or Deadly Doctrine by Harold Koenig

The Soul in Distress: What Every Pastoral Counselor Should Know About Emotional and Mental Illness by Richard Roukema

Pastoral Care
in Pregnancy Loss
A Ministry Long Needed

Thomas Moe, DMin

The Haworth Pastoral Press
An Imprint of The Haworth Press, Inc.
New York • London

Published by

The Haworth Pastoral Press, an imprint of The Haworth Press, Inc., 10 Alice Street, Binghamton, NY 13904-1580

Cover design by Marylouise E. Doyle.

Scripture taken from the *Holy Bible, New International Version*©. Copyright © 1973, 1978, 1984 by International Bible Society. Used by permission of International Bible Society.
"*NIV*" and "*New International Version*" are trademarks registered in the United States Patent and Trademark office by International Bible Society.

Library of Congress Cataloging-in-Publication Data

Moe, Thomas.
    Pastoral care in pregnancy loss : a ministry long needed / Thomas Moe.
      p.   cm.
    Includes bibliographical references (p.   ) and index.
    ISBN 0-7890-0124-1 (alk. paper)
    1. Women–Pastoral counseling of. 2. Miscarriage–Religious aspects–Christianity. I. Title.
BV4445.M64 1997
259'.6–dc20

                                               96-9343
                                               CIP

To Brian James Moe
Born and died July 6, 1980
Some people come into our lives
and we are never ever the same
From Mom, Dad, Elisabeth, Cynthia
and Eric.

ABOUT THE AUTHOR

Thomas Moe, DMin, is an ordained minister serving in the United Methodist Church. Dr. Moe has been a consultant to several organizations providing care to individuals experiencing pregnancy loss, including RTS Bereavement Services, a hospital-based program specializing in providing multidisciplinary care for those who have experienced pregnancy loss. Since its beginning in 1981, this program has expanded to over 100 units worldwide. Dr. Moe received his Doctor of Ministry degree from Bethel Theological Seminary with a specialty in pregnancy loss ministry and has led numerous clergy seminars on the subject.

CONTENTS

Preface

Many a church leader will, at first, cringe at the thought of a book such as this. After all, most church leaders already have more than enough to do. Their schedules are well filled with existing programs. Very likely, their churches struggle to provide the resources to maintain these existing programs. The thought of adding another program of ministry will not be immediately welcomed by these folks.

My purpose is not just to add more stress to the existing program life of a church. Instead, this writing intends to help the church focus upon the people in its midst who suffer hurt from pregnancy loss. These people are a part of almost every church. Yet, most faith communities could not be less prepared to meet their needs and deal with their hurt. The leadership in most churches do not know how to provide even basic ministry to these people. Instead, these individuals tend to travel from church to church, staying long enough to exhaust resources but seldom finding a ministry of help. It is my hope that churches and other faith communities will begin to understand those who have experienced grief from pregnancy loss and to learn means of effective ministry to them. With this understanding, faith communities will be able to help these bereaved persons work through their grief and grow in the resolution process. Instead of church members and leaders feeling inadequate as they watch these grievers continually traveling from location to location for ministry, a church can grow with them as resolution takes form.

Hopefully, the reader will understand that this ministry requires more effort than simply setting up another program within the church. While such a program can be very helpful, it often merely isolates the churches from feeling the experiences of their people. This writing wishes to help the church transcend programming to enter the world of those who grieve from pregnancy loss. Like the busy priests and Levites of a too-familiar parable, many of us have been able to walk by the sufferers of pregnancy loss and not notice the suffering. This book attempts to move us into the role of Samaritans who can actually stop, experience the suffering, and nurture healing.

I would like to thank my loving family for their support and encouragement in this writing. I am extremely grateful to the many caring people who have given of their time and expertise, which allows me to present this information to you. My special appreciation goes to those individuals who have allowed their experiences in pregnancy loss to become the living documents that you may now study. While their identity has been hidden from you, I hope that in some way the lives so greatly missed by many may live in our minds as we expand our scope of ministry.

Acknowledgment

I would like to acknowledge the past and present staff of Bereavement Services RTS at Gundersen Lutheran Medical Center, Wisconsin. They truly are people who know how to care.

Chapter 1

Pregnancy Loss Ministry

UNDERSTANDING THE PROBLEM

Most religious leaders today do not mean to be insensitive to those suffering from pregnancy loss. Unlike the religious leaders in the Good Samaritan parable who saw suffering and ignored its victims, most church leaders today are caring people who do not minister because they are completely unaware that any suffering is involved with a pregnancy loss. They may see the symptoms of suffering and grief but never understand that actual suffering and grief are taking place. This has happened for a number of reasons. I highlight two major ones.

The first reason that the church is not adequately ministering to those suffering from pregnancy loss is that we have bought into the American success myth. In this success myth, one assumes that the death of a baby is an extremely rare occurrence. This makes sense to many since America has some of the world's best health care facilities and some of the world's most health-conscious people. Therefore, many assume that America is unlike other lesser developed countries where the death of a baby can be a frequent event.

This view of America and American health care is far from reality. America, while ahead of many other nations in the quality of health care, remains behind most industrial nations in all forms of infant survival rate. The number of babies who die from pregnancy loss every year is unusually high. While it is difficult to obtain accurate data, a consistent pattern has remained over the recent decades: approximately only three-fourths of all conceptions actually create a living baby. Some statistics indicate an even higher rate of pregnancy loss, perhaps as high as 50 percent or even higher.[1]

Statistical accuracy is difficult because many of the miscarriages occur so early in the pregnancy that the mother is unaware of the miscarriage. She may think that menstruation is late, and when the miscarriage occurs it is just "unusually heavy"; thus, she does not even recognize the loss. Whatever the actual statistic, it is clear that a large number of pregnancies in America every year will not come to term. Many of these losses will leave the bereaved family devastated. This book will focus upon three types of these losses: miscarriage, stillbirth, and neonatal loss, and the ministries that can be helpful to those who experience these tragedies.

For too long the church has lived in the myth of successful American health care. We have not entered into a deliberate style of ministry to those suffering from pregnancy loss because we have not been aware of the problem's magnitude. The task of the contemporary church requires that we move from our world of myth to one that faces reality. Reality will force us to minister among those people who hurt from these tragedies. In setting up these ministries, the church must also develop a strategy for fulfilling such ministry. Simply put, we must avoid letting the American success myth limit the scope of our ministry. By understanding the magnitude of the loss, we will be compelled to find ways in which we can respond with quality ministry.

The second reason that the church has not played the role of a Good Samaritan to those suffering from pregnancy loss is our ignorance that victims of pregnancy loss may be truly grieving. There are so many ways to avoid seeing people grieving from pregnancy loss. By not seeing any hurt, we have convinced ourselves that our distortions are the reality. These distortions have been around for some time. As for the disciples of Matthew 19:13-15, our world often minimizes the small child as "lesser" than a grown child. Sometimes the parents who have suffered pregnancy loss will also help enforce that distortion by pretending that they do not experience hurt. Our world will encourage them "to get on with their life," or assure them, "that they can have another," and encourage them to cover their grief with meaningless clichés. For pastoral caregivers who become aware that grief may be occurring in those who suffer from pregnancy loss, ministry is often withheld assuming that "the needs are mostly medical and hospital or medical staff will care for all that."

In reality, pregnancy loss includes emotional grief and suffering. It creates many spiritual problems. As church leaders we overestimate the possibilities of health care being able to touch and meet the needs of people affected by such grief and suffering. While medical personnel are caring people, most have enough responsibility in meeting the physical needs of patients without ministering to their deeper emotional needs. All of this causes the griever suffering from pregnancy loss to "fall between the cracks" of the support systems.

Even in the best of settings, the church has generally understated the effects of grief upon human life. Research is just beginning to see how grief affects the entire person. Unresolved grief is being traced as a root problem in numerous significant illnesses, including cancer, compulsive behavior disorders, and many emotional disorders. Research in 1944 by Erich Lindemann found that mourners can be at risk for:

> some seven deadly diseases including heart attack, high blood pressure, cancer, skin diseases, rheumatoid arthritis, diabetes, and thyroid malfunction. Others have added numbers of emotional disorders, compulsive disorders, and many various chronic "aches and pains."[2]

These illnesses can result from pregnancy loss as well as any other type of grief. We can only speculate as to other possible results of such loss.

Perhaps a tragic irony can be found that all of this ignorance is occurring during the time of the abortion crisis, which should be bringing significant focus upon the worth of the unborn and the rights of parents to make choices. Ironically, in spite of all the concern that has come from the issues regarding induced abortion, little focus has moved to compassion for those who have experienced pregnancy loss.

TYPES OF PREGNANCY LOSS

The following is a general explanation of the three types of pregnancy losses:

1. *Miscarriage* is, by far, the most frequent cause of pregnancy loss. While actual definition may vary with different medical organizations, a miscarriage is often described as a pregnancy loss that occurs before twenty weeks of gestation. A baby born dead after twenty weeks of gestation is often referred to as a stillbirth. Miscarriage may sometimes be referred as a "spontaneous abortion." Miscarriage is overwhelmingly the most frequent among all types of pregnancy loss, accounting for some 95 percent of such losses. Again, while accurate statistics are difficult to obtain, it is believed that at least 15-25 percent of all conceptions will end in a miscarriage. Some consider these statistics quite conservative. The vast majority of these miscarriages will be so early in the pregnancy that the mother is not even aware that the pregnancy ever occurred.

2. *Stillbirth* is another type of loss that can occur during a pregnancy. In stillbirth, the baby is born dead. It is estimated that perhaps as little as under 1 percent of all conceptions terminate in stillbirth. While this number appears small, it is important to note that there may be over 30,000 such losses in America each year. That will be three times the equivalent of the number of annual losses to Sudden Infant Death Syndrome (SIDS). In spite of the equal frequency, the church is much more equipped and available to sympathize with those experiencing the latter loss than those experiencing stillbirth, or any other form of pregnancy loss.

3. *Newborn death* is a death of a baby within the first month of birth. It is often referred to as "neonatal loss." Newborn loss usually results from a difficulty during gestation, such as lack of organ development. Each year in the United States there are approximately 35,000 newborn deaths.

4. *Other pregnancy losses* can occur due to problems such as ectopic pregnancy, in which the embryo has not attached to a part of the uterus that can support the life of the baby. An "incompetent cervix," where the uterus cannot hold the fertilized egg, can also lead to a loss. There are other less common forms of pregnancy loss that can be better explained in resources found in the bibliography.

A final type of pregnancy loss, *induced abortion,* will not be included in this study. Induced abortion occurs when a pregnancy is medically terminated. While this book can be helpful in ministry to those who have had an induced abortion, this form of pregnancy loss may create entirely different sorts of problems that are greater than the capacities of this writing.

THE NATIONAL PROBLEM

The fact that the United States has a large number of baby losses comes as a surprise to most people. Yet, it is a fact. America has continually been a per capita leader in many different types of baby losses compared to other industrialized nations. Most countries do not keep an accurate record of miscarriages and stillbirths. It is difficult, then, to get accurate statistics to discover how the United States actually compares to these countries. However, The World Health Organization has kept accurate statistics in infant mortality across the world.[3] Their statistics indicate that the United States has significantly more infant losses than other nations of similar economic strength. Table 1.1 lists some statistical examples.

One notes that the United States ranks very high in infant mortality compared to other nations around the world. Even with our much superior health care, we still rank behind Canada in preventing infant mortality per live births. Our slower improvement rate over the past twenty years has allowed nations such as Spain, Israel, and even Taiwan to pass the United States. While the United States still ranks significantly higher than lesser economically developed coun-

Table 1.1
Infant Mortality Per 1,000 Live Births (3)

Nation	Year: 1977/8	1994	1995
Taiwan	18.0	6	5.6
Israel	17.8	9	7.0
Spain	15.6	7	7.6
United States	14.0	10	8.3
Australia	12.5	7	6.1
Canada	12.2	7	7.0
Japan	8.9	4	4.4
Sweden	7.7	6	4.8

tries such as Mexico, which recorded 27 infant deaths per 1,000 live births in 1994, the gap is being quickly closed. Even the new war-torn nation of Croatia had lower infant mortality rates in 1994 than did the United States.

It is difficult to understand why these numbers are so out of proportion to our economic and medical development compared to other nations in the world. It is even more difficult to explain our inability to solve the dilemma. Some will argue that specific geographic pockets of our population where poor health care is the rule may make these statistics look unusually high. However, other nations also may have certain such pockets that should keep their statistics high as well. Others will argue that there is a connection between our advancing pollution and our high rate of loss.

Unfortunately, no one can give a clear answer for the problem. Until we discover the reason, we will not be able to take measures to solve the problem, assuming a solution is possible. Even if we were able to give a reason for these losses, it would never ease the grief of the many families who have suffered through these horrendous experiences of losing their babies.

The problem for most pastors or church members is more than a lack of awareness of the amount of pregnancy losses that may occur in their congregation. Very few of us are aware of the impact these losses can have upon grievers. Most of the general public still thinks of pregnancy loss as a lesser loss than a loss of a "child that really lived." The reasoning appears to follow this pattern. Expecting parents have had little contact with their child. This is particularly so compared to parents who have had their child for many years. Less contact should mean less acute levels of grief. Therefore, a parent of a twelve-year-old who died would have more grief that a parent of a four-year-old who died. That same parent of a four-year-old would have more grief, the logic follows, than the parent of a deceased baby. Our "scale" would go down to parents of a newborn who has died having more grief than parents suffering from stillbirth loss, who would have more grief than parents grieving a miscarriage loss. All of these losses, according to the theory, would involve less grief than the loss of a twenty-year-old child. This value system has been given near universal acceptance in our culture.

THE MINISTRY PROBLEM

Unfortunately, the value system described above is based upon the experiences of outside observers of loss rather than through the experiences of the parent. This is because we, as clergy or church members, will have had little experience with an unborn child who is a part of another family. We usually will have no awareness of another couple's experiences as they anticipate their new child. We seldom will closely interact with the anticipation of the baby once the pregnancy is determined. We never will experience morning sickness, the fetal movement, or the other changes in body and lifestyle that come from the pregnancy and lead to daily and hourly reminders of the baby. Without these continued reminders, we do not develop attachment to the baby at a level similar to the parent, especially similar to the expecting mother. Without these experiences that affirm the anticipation of birth, we are not able to develop any sense of hope for or attachment to the child. Some close friends may develop limited attachment but none will understand the attachment of the family. In contrast to the distancing others will experience, a study by Kennell and Klause indicated that many parents begin intimate emotional attachment very early in the pregnancy.[4] For those with only limited involvement and attachment, there will also be limited feeling of grief if the pregnancy comes to a tragic end. Without an understanding of family attachment, grief makes little sense. For those who have not developed an understanding of the grief, the grief of the family does not make sense. All too often, if we do not feel or understand the grief, we then assume that the parents do not either. Unfortunately, that assumption is generally false.

This false assumption leads to further problems in our care of families grieving from pregnancy loss. Since we have had little personal experience with the loss, we benefit by not developing any emotional attachments to those who are feeling the pregnancy loss. We will not want to think–let alone talk–about the deceased child because it will make us experience the child and will create grief for us. We do not provide an opportunity for the family to have our ministry resources because this experience will create pain for ourselves.

Many clergy will physically be present for a pastoral call when there is a pregnancy loss, but will not enter into the emotional experience of the family. This leaves the family alone to find their way through the grief experience.

> Some priests, ministers, and rabbis compound the situation by setting themselves above grief and tears, either as an example of fortitude or for self protection. A greater problem is that most members of the clergy receive little training in bereavement counseling during their formal education. Divinity students who wish to become hospital chaplains are the most likely to have bereavement training, but their exposure to pregnancy loss and infant death may still be minimal. This lack of preparation can leave members of the clergy so out of touch with the needs of bereaved parents that they may make errors of judgment and taste.[5]

Even further, many well-intentioned people, including clergy, will feel that they are doing a service to the grieving family by helping to remove the experience of the pregnancy loss. Some may try to minimize the loss by treating the baby as an object that was less than human. Some may even refuse to discuss the subject with the family. Others, well-intended in ministry, can be incredibly clandestine, including entering the home and removing all baby items "before Mom comes home from the hospital to see them." All of this serves to distance the parent from helpful support systems.

Studies, mostly since the 1970s, show that intensity of parental grief does not follow any sliding scales based upon the age of the deceased child. Among others, Zahourek and Jensen show that grief can show more intensity among those who have suffered a miscarriage over those who have had a born child die.[6] Herz indicates that families will bond to unborn children and will develop strong ties that will result in significant grief.[7] Benfield, Leib, and Vollman indicate that the grief from newborn death has no connection with the size of the baby or duration of his or her life.[8]These studies indicate that our old value system has long been in need of a change.

Some of these changes require more than simply a change of attitude. There are official church doctrines that influence our ministry. For example, the Roman Catholic Church had long held to the doctrine of an eternal state of limbo for those who have died in pregnancy or before a baptism has been made available to them.

This doctrine has traditionally created some difficulties for ministry to the surviving family. The deceased child is lowered to a state something less than a full human and, therefore, not in need of the ministry of the church. Adding further to the problem, the doctrine teaches grieving parents that they will have little hope of ever meeting that child in eternity. Further, the child would be separated from the face of God "forever." There is nothing that a parent can do for that child to get that person into heaven since baptism is not an option for children either born deceased or having died before the ritual could be administered. This doctrine adds to the grief of the family members by adding to their sense of failure in providing a successful pregnancy. The doctrine of limbo has limited the ministries, such as funeral ministries, available to the family coping with loss, since the child will not have been baptized, he or she is ineligible for such ministry. In many ways, regarding pregnancy loss, the door of ministry is officially closed for those adhering to this doctrine.

Many will argue that, since Vatican II, significant changes have occurred that allow for new opportunities for ministry in the Roman Catholic Church. While not directly a part of Vatican II, the doctrines of limbo have also been significantly altered subsequent to that event. However, Vatican II and its implications have not yet fully impacted upon many individual parishes in the Roman Catholic Church, leaving many parishoners dealing with the traditional dilemma. Even in parishes where Vatican II has been fully implemented, there are often many who still hold to pre-Vatican values, which may lead to the continued problem.

Other religious beliefs can create similar difficulties. For example, according to the Talmud, many in the Jewish tradition do not allow funerals for children who died within the first month of life. This is carried out particularly among the followers of Orthodox faith. The Reformed Jewish faith places an option for such care in the hands of the particular rabbi. The door of ministry is officially closed in practice, however, when the family wishes to have the child of pregnancy loss buried in the cemetery of their faith.

Faith communities are not the only institutions with policies that limit the care provided for families suffering from pregnancy loss. Funeral directors will often strongly discourage funerals after pregnancy loss. Some funeral directors have a policy of providing only private graveside rites for small children. Traditionally, this was to avoid causing "difficulty" for others by involving them in the grieving process.

Medical institutions can also have an official policy that hinders the ability to care for individuals suffering from a pregnancy loss. Many hospitals limit parents from any contact with babies who were miscarried or died at or shortly after birth. Medical records will often refer to the miscarriage as "spontaneous abortion" assuming that the patient will recognize the difference between a spontaneous abortion (miscarriage) and an induced abortion (with intention). For some, the terminology can add a terrible implication to the already painful experience.

Clergy insensitivity can occur in many forms. Unfortunately, most clergy are blind to their insensitivity. Most clergy would indicate that they provide strong support for those who have undergone bereavement. Few would indicate that they had a bias against any form of bereavement. However, a study performed at Lutheran Hospital in La Crosse, Wisconsin showed otherwise. In a study of 284 area clergy of numerous denominations, it was shown that clergy are significantly less likely to respond in ministry when there is a pregnancy loss compared to another form of loss such as the death of a younger child, a teen, or a young adult.[9] In case studies, either grief from the loss or ministry for the grief was considered inappropriate when the loss was:

Given the same setting, clergy were actually five times more likely to consider the loss not deserving of ministry if it were a miscarriage loss compared to the loss of a 12-year-old. In this study, there was a slow increase of available ministry as the age of the

Table 1.2
Clergy Response to Loss Based on Age of Child

TYPE OF LOSS	TIMES CONSIDERED NOT WORTHY OF MINISTRY:
Miscarriage	70 times of 284 or 24.6% of respondents
Baby	29 times of 284 or 10.2% of respondents
4-year-old	18 times of 284 or 6.3% of respondents
12-year-old	14 times of 284 or 4.9% of respondents

deceased child increased. Even more troubling were the clergy comments in the study toward the losses. Not only did some clergy show insensitivity toward pregnancy loss, but some also indicated that any such parental grief had little place in the Christian life.

Such insensitivity adds to the grief of the family who has undergone pregnancy loss. While the statistical data is very unclear regarding the impact of loss upon the family, most family therapists see such loss as a significant problem. In her classic text, *Parental Loss of a Child*, Therese Rando brings the problem to the forefront by stating,

> All of these secondary losses place additional burdens of grief, loss and adaptation on couples already overwrought with responsibilities and demands. These problems contribute to the assertion that there may be higher divorce rates in bereaved couples. However, it is invalid to assume that the loss of a child must lead to parental divorce.[10]

While attempting to be optimistic, Rando does not portray a positive setting. She indicates the nature of the problem in hoping that family therapists will not automatically assume that the relationship is doomed. The meaning hidden beneath her words is that the loss of a child can be devastating to a marriage relationship. There are a number of books that can chronicle these relational problems. Some of these books can be found in the bibliography. *When a Baby Dies* by Rana K. Limbo and Sara Rich Wheeler can identify the issues extremely well in a short amount of reading.

While researchers indicate that some marriages may grow stronger as a result of the grieving, it is too optimistic to assume that it will happen in any given case. Even if true, we would not use that assumption for any other setting. For example, knowing a that break in a bone may cause a healing that creates a stronger bone is little help to the suffering victim. Such optimism is no substitute for emergency medical care. In the same manner, the church needs to be aware of the considerable problems that pregnancy loss may place upon a family. The hope that a relationship may grow stronger is no substitute for emergency care.

Family crisis from pregnancy loss comes in many forms, not only marital. It may be in relationship difficulties between the father and mother. It may be in planning for future pregnancies. It may be in responding to the needs of the grandparents of the deceased. It may be in overprotecting other children or trying to replace the lost child. In time, all of these issues may pose significant problems for the family. In the next chapters, specific stories will illustrate some of these difficulties.

It is my belief that this study will be beneficial to everyone involved in ministry. Without a doubt, it has to be the most difficult area of ministry to study. Among other difficulties, the study is emotionally taxing. In my doctoral thesis involving case studies of individuals and couples who had experienced pregnancy loss, each interview left me feeling emotionally exhausted. Early on, as I began to set up further meetings, I learned not to schedule two interviews without an extended break in-between. I needed the time to recover from one interview before taking on another. Yet, while the work was long, tedious, and sometimes extremely painful, the study of pregnancy loss brought to me a reality of the major issues of life, including but not only the shortness of time on earth, relationships of God and suffering, living with apparent injustices, and discovering the purpose of life. I hope the study will do the same for you. While it did not give me the answers, it has helped me form the questions. This is because the issues of pregnancy loss lead us to the heart of all of life issues. Some of the most unanswerable questions of life come from pregnancy loss. Those who are able to minister in such a setting become better able to minister in many other difficult settings. It follows the pattern of the parable, "To those who have much, more will be given." For too long many of us have avoided the things that these issues can give to us. It is no consolation to know that this lack of understanding in ministry is not just an American problem. It is a flaw of ministry worldwide. While little research is taking place to identify the scope of the problem, churches in other countries may even be behind those in the United States:

> No pastoral visits in the local parish with direct connection to the perinatal loss have been reported when it concerns the Church of Sweden.[11]

In spite of these trends, faith communities remain the most appropriate place to face these issues and find a hope that comes from God. In our society, many medical personnel, funeral directors, and grief sufferers around us are hoping that we, the church, can add direction in support to those who are experiencing this loss. It is my hope that your faith community becomes equipped to provide this ministry rather than to expect that another discipline will take our task upon themselves. If that be your goal as well, this book will serve you well toward that quest.

NOTES

1. Ilse, S., and L.H. Burns. *Miscarriage: A Shattered Dream.* Burnsville, NC: Rainbow Connection, 1989.

2. Davidson, G.W. *Understanding Mourning.* Minneapolis: Augsburg Press, 1984.

3. World Health Organization reports found in Annual World Almanacs.

4. Kohn, I., and P. Moffitt. *A Silent Sorrow: Pregnancy Loss.* New York: Delacorte Press, Bantam Doubleday Dell Publishing Group, 1992, p. 6.

5. Kohn, I., and P. Moffitt. *A Silent Sorrow: Pregnancy Loss.* New York: Delacorte Press, Bantam Doubleday Dell Publishing, 1992, p. 190.

6. Zahourek, R., and J. Jensen. "Grieving and the Loss of a Newborn, " *American Journal of Nursing,* 73, (May, 1973): 836-839.

7. Herz, F. The Impact of Death and Serious Illness on the Family Life Cycle. In E. Carter and M. McGoldrick (Eds.), *The Family Life Cycle.* New York: Gardner.

8. Benfield, D.G., S.A. Leib, and J.H. Vollman. "Grief Responses of Parents to Neonatal Death and Parent Participation in Deciding Care." *Pediatrics,* 62 (1978): 171-177.

9. Moe, T. *Ministry to Families Suffering from Loss Due to Miscarriage, Stillbirth, or Neonatal Death.* Doctoral thesis, Bethel Theological Seminary, St. Paul, MN, 1993.

10. Rando, T.A. *Parental Loss of a Child.* Champaign, IL: Research Press, 1986, p. 29.

11. Wretmark, A.A. *Perinatal Death as a Pastoral Problem.* Uppsala, Sweden: Bibliotheca Theologiae Practicae, 1993, p. 15; as quoted by K.F. Finckling in *Journal of Pastoral Care* (Fall 1995): 344-346.

Chapter 2

Case Studies in Pregnancy Loss

CASE STUDY ONE: CAN'T COME TO CHURCH

Steve and Toni, a bright young couple in an otherwise aging rural church, have had two children. They attend church regularly. Toni's parents and grandparents have attended this same church and have been very active in its ministry for many years. Steve has not had a long history of involvement in the life of a church. Since joining Toni's church, Steve has enjoined becoming active in leadership positions. This is unlike most younger families of Toni's church. For various reasons, most of the younger generation in the church no longer attend. Not only are Steve and Toni known as the members of the younger generation that have not left, their enthusiasm has also been marvelous in attracting new families to the church. Steve and Toni have been extremely helpful in giving hope to an aging congregation.

When it was announced that Steve and Toni were expecting their third child, the entire church celebrated with all of Toni's extended family. However, two months into the pregnancy, Toni began spotting blood. A day later she miscarried. The pastor did not know about the miscarriage until worship the next Sunday when Toni's name was mentioned in a prayer request. He felt a bit awkward in that most of the congregation seemed to already know about the loss.

That afternoon the pastor visited Steve and Toni's home. Steve seemed to be in reasonably good spirits and was able to express gratitude that he was blessed with two wonderful children and a good wife. Steve seemed to be relieved that things were not worse. The physicians expressed a bit of concern about Toni during the miscarriage. Steve was relieved that she could come home so soon.

Toni was not able to speak very much with the pastor. She came out of the bedroom where she had been sleeping all day. Steve indicated that Toni had been feeling this way since the miscarriage three days earlier, but indicated that the physicians hoped that she would be "over it soon." The pastor had prayer before Toni went back to bed. After a short conversation with Steve, the pastor left.

In two weeks Toni was able to go back to work. Because of financial pressures, she began working full-time rather than the doctor's recommendation of part-time. At first, the pastor was not concerned that Toni and Steve were not coming back to church. He called on occasion to hear Steve assure him that things were coming along, "slow but ok." It seemed a bit odd to the pastor to only talk with Steve. In the past, Toni had always answered the telephone. However, he dismissed his concerns as did others in the church who knew Toni quite well, and he reinforced Steve's positive expectation. The pastor was able to justify Toni's sudden lack of interest in the church. Certainly, Toni had a lot of demands upon her and she needed to take time to rest rather than come to church. He hoped things would be different in a short time.

Three months later things were different but not as the pastor had hoped. Toni had not been at church and Steve and the children were also frequently absent. The church members were feeling the loss and becoming very uneasy. There was concern that this could develop into something very serious for the church. Everyone there knew that no one else was able to attract younger families the way that Steve and Toni were able to do so. Without Toni, Steve and the children didn't seem as interested in attending.

This was addressed as a major concern at the very next administrative council meeting. Vacation Bible School plans were due to begin. Toni had always cared for the VBS leadership work. Without Toni, the Bible School would be in serious risk of cancellation. Of even greater concern to the administrative council, reports were circulating that Steve and Toni had been "trying out" other churches in a nearby community. There was concern that perhaps the pastor had not provided enough ministry to Steve and Toni. With all at stake, the administrative council insisted that the pastor make a visit and that he report back immediately.

The pastor, given the directive, made plans to visit with Steve and Toni the next day. Upon entering their home, he noted that the setting was much the same as his first visit shortly after hearing of the miscarriage. Toni seemed very depressed and not interested in talking. Steve seemed unaware that much was wrong and, as during the first visit, assured the pastor that Toni would get over the problem in a short time. Steve appeared quite apologetic for her state.

In this and the series of visits in the following weeks, the pastor kept inviting Steve and Toni to return to church as soon as possible. Both Steve and Toni expressed interest in returning. The pastor seemed comfortable in preparing to report to the administrative council that things were "falling into place." Though it appeared that Toni would not be able to provide leadership for this year's Bible School, things would be better next year.

On the day of the next administrative council meeting, Toni called the pastor. She seemed very bitter as she informed the pastor that she and her family would be going to another church in another community and would want their membership removed from the church. Shocked, the pastor wondered, "What was wrong? How had they failed? What would he tell the administrative council?"

Pastoral Issues

A number of pastoral issues occurred in this account. The first issue is the problem that Peppers and Knapp refer to as incongruent grieving.[1] This will be covered in more detail in Chapter 5.

The second issue involves a lack of understanding toward pregnancy loss. At the time of pregnancy loss, a physician may have had little attachment to the pregnancy, perhaps becoming involved for the first time in an emergency center as the pregnancy loss takes place. In Toni's case, the physician had no grief experience in the loss and saw little need for her to experience emotional trauma. While, medically speaking Toni was all right, the physician was not able to see the whole picture. The physician did not see that pregnancy loss involves issues that transcend any one level of professional expertise. He did not understand that no one can readily predict the emotional impact that trauma can place upon an individual.

While most physicians are caring persons who attempt to understand the emotional and spiritual needs of the patient as well as their physical needs, they are not able to predict the future. When a physician attempts to identify all solutions of human need within his or her expertise, others need to find appropriate ways to question that judgment. Unfortunately, Steve also agreed with the physician and never understood the depth of Toni's trauma.

The pastor experienced a number of common problems in his ministry with Steve and Toni's church. Like so many others in pastoral ministry have experienced, he was never in the "information circle" of the church that he served. He found himself "in the dark" regarding Steve and Toni's loss and had to "catch up" when he heard of the miscarriage long after she had come home from the hospital. However, the problems worsened as the church showed complete inability to minister to the needs of the family. They were more concerned about Steve and Toni's ability to serve them than they were concerned about Steve and Toni as people. The church showed a problem similar to many churches in desiring to maintain their "status quo" without regard to effective and caring ministry. They really were not concerned that Steve and Toni did not attend church. They only expressed concern when Steve and Toni were rumored to be receiving ministry elsewhere. The problem became messier as the administrative council placed guilt upon the pastor for not "ministering properly." The concern was totally for the institution of the church. Unfortunately, the pastor bought into that mandate and, predictably, failed miserably in ministry.

There are many issues that might lead to Toni's distancing herself from the church after her loss. For example, Toni may have experienced church in the framework of her family setting. Since her childhood years, Toni may have been in the building with her parents and grandparents. In recent years, she had been attending with her husband and children. Everything about the church had reminded her of her family. Unfortunately, after a pregnancy loss, her immediate thoughts of her family were not pleasant. The church would serve as a monument to her that her family was no longer intact. With this in mind, it is easy to understand why people such as Toni, suffering from the loss of a child, find it difficult to attend their home church.

For most people, death occurs with little or no meaning. This is especially true for death due to pregnancy loss. Often, the couple will be required to wait from four to six weeks for the medical reports to be completed following a pregnancy loss. The process of waiting for information from these medical reports can be long and taxing. Often, waiting for the reports only presents a false hope to the couple that they will have any medical answers for their loss.

> The fact that physicians are not able to determine a cause in over 50 percent of miscarriages can be enormously frustrating, especially if you have endured weeks or months of testing. When you do not know the cause of your pregnancy loss, you also lack a specific course to follow in trying to prevent a subsequent miscarriage, so that succeeding pregnancies may be fraught with uncertainty and anxiety.[2]

For people such as Steve and Toni, there is little to explain, to provide meaning, or to justify the loss. Bereaved parents such as Steve and Toni may seek to create meanings. Very often other "Steve and Tonis" will discover a meaning of their loss in a lack of blessing. Much like the mother in the next case study, they will stay away from church because they feel uncomfortable in a setting where their lack of blessing may be magnified. Often, they will not be able to express their feelings but, instead, will give excuses for their continued absence from the church.

Churches that are desperate for "warm bodies" will place all sorts of pressures upon people such as Toni to return into the active status of the church. They may often lack any form of tact in so doing. At first, someone like Toni may feel comfortable in confabulating reasons why she cannot attend and serve. Eventually, these reasons will run out, and she will be confronted with a demand to return. This will often come in some form of a guilt-inducement request. As the administrative council put guilt upon the pastor, so they will put the same guilt upon Steve and Toni. The people of the church do not mean to cause harm, they merely use guilt as a survival tact. Unfortunately, neither they nor Steve and Toni end up surviving the relationship. Eventually, Steve and Toni must face the confrontation. The results usually are tragic for the church relationship. Instead of facing their difficulty, they remove their membership from the church and sever the ties from the group that is most likely to provide them with the long-term support and understanding that their grieving needs. Adding to the problem, if Toni is struggling with feelings of lack in blessing, changing churches will do little to help her problem. Often people such as Toni will attempt to find other churches only to discover a double grief: they still experience the lack of their blessing and add grief by experiencing a loss of their church home.

Ministry could have occurred in a number of ways. First, the church focus needed to move from the institution of the church to the people of the church. This is not a simple step. If the church could not make that step, the pastor or another leader needed to take appropriate action. However, many church leaders tend to focus on the institution of the church as a priority. They can even prevent the type of care that Steve and Toni needed from happening. This church did so by continually placing the pastor in a defensive position rather than by allowing him any control to develop effective ministry. They started him off "in the dark" by not informing him of the miscarriage. They controlled his ministry scope with their clear goal: "Get Steve and Toni back into church." Had any of the parties been able to focus on Toni, her needs may have been discovered and a supportive setting could allow for her healing. Unfortunately, too often this never happens.

A final issue often enters into settings such as these. The physician, the pastor, and Steve all entered into a false hope that time would solve Toni's problems. Grief seldom works that way. Time may make the pain less sharp. However, after the sharpness of the pain subsides, often the bitterness remains. Rather than push one through a grief process such as all ended doing to Toni, it is wise to allow individuals to take their time until they feel "ready" to return to past lifestyles.

> Throw deadlines out the window. Don't place expectations on yourself to feel better after a certain amount of time. Give yourself permission to feel your feelings, to feel bad and to start feeling better whenever that occurs.
>
> Remember that grief has its ups and downs, and you will feel discouraged when you have setbacks. You deserve all the time you need. Do what is best for you, what you need to do to cope with your baby's death.[3]

To assume that one will have the same grief experience as another or that there is an average time for grief is to not understand the uniqueness of attachment and grief loss. People will have unique styles that require unique ministries. It would be like assuming that since size ten is an average size shoe everyone ought to wear shoes as close to a size ten as possible. As people need to wear shoes that fit their feet, so they need to grieve in a way that fits their feeling of loss. In ministry, we need to help that happen.

CASE STUDY TWO: "I FAILED GOD"

Recently things have been difficult for Mike and Susan. They had been facing unusual financial pressures. In addition, for a significant amount of time other pressures had been building upon their relationship because Susan had difficulty becoming pregnant. After expensive testing it had been determined that Susan's difficulty was a problem with her ovulation. With more expensive treatment and patient waiting, things changed. Mike and Susan were so happy when they announced at Mike's family Thanksgiving gathering that they would be expecting their first child in late spring.

While Mike and Susan anticipated the joy in their family, they had no idea how much excitement the announcement would actually create. Large families were a tradition in Mike's home. Mike's father came from a large family; he was the only boy among seven sisters. Mike also was the only son among four older sisters. With few sons, there was concern that the family name might be lost. It was now up to Mike and Susan to carry on the family name as his father and mother did when they had their fifth child.

The Thanksgiving dinner suddenly became a time of great celebration. Even Mike's brothers-in-law got into the act. All were in happy spirits. Some of it seemed a little too personal for Susan, but since she was among family she found the touching of her tummy by all the relatives acceptable and eventually began to enjoy the attention. "Mike and I have waited a long time for this child and we deserve all the enjoyment of the holiday," she reasoned. The celebration reached a crescendo after the evening dishes were done when Mike announced that he was taking Susan home to be sure that she got plenty of rest. As they were going out the door, Mike's grandfather hugged Susan and gave her the family blessing. Her mother-in-law had tears in her eyes as she, too, hugged her and said, "I'm so glad you are not like other girls who won't fulfill their obligation."

With such expectations, everything should have been fine and Susan should have nothing to give her concern. However, the family financial status was far from good. To make matters worse, Mike and Susan were struggling to make their monthly payments for their house. Sometimes the struggle lead to conflict. The expected baby brought unusual tension to the situation. Conflict between Mike and Susan seemed to be reaching a peak just before Thanksgiving.

Within a week of their wonderful Thanksgiving, Mike and Susan got into a terrible fight in their upstairs bedroom regarding Susan's use of a charge card. Susan suddenly heard words blurt out at Mike that she couldn't believe were from her. Embarrassed, she turned to go downstairs. In her upset state, Susan tripped and fell down several steps. Mike forgot the argument as he came to Susan's rescue. He was visibly shaken even though Susan insisted that she was not hurt. A week later she began to spot blood. In a short time she miscarried.

Suddenly, their joy turned into devastation. Susan began to feel that she had let her entire family down. Susan began looking for causes to the disaster. She began to reason to herself, "If only I did not make Mike angry by such careless use of the charge card. If only I had not lost control of myself and said those horrible things to Mike. If only I wasn't so clumsy and tripped on those stairs. I could have avoided the miscarriage."

Even though her obstetrician assured her that there was no connection between her miscarriage and these events, she was certain they were connected. Further, she felt guilty about her inability to ovulate properly. "If not for my problems," she thought, "Mike could have plenty of children." As the days passed, Susan even wondered if Mike would have been better off if he had married someone else. Perhaps even anyone else.

Susan's guilt continued to grow day by day. Adding to her problems, the gynecologist delivered even worse news a week later. Because of her age and progressive difficulty in ovulation, the gynecologist insisted that another pregnancy was less than realistic.

In a short time Mike and Susan would gather again with Mike's family, this time for Christmas dinner. As she anticipated the event, Susan worried, "How can I face Mike's family? What can I say? God has given me everything I ever thought I wanted in a supportive family. My husband tries hard to care for me. Why couldn't I reward them with a son?"

Adding to her self blame, Mike and Susan had most recently undergone infertility testing. The results of that test had recently arrived and they indicated quite clearly that his sperm count was not the problem. The infertility was clearly the result of her ovulation difficulty. While the physicians tried to not specifically state it as such, Susan left the consultation with the clear understanding that she was the problem.

"When I finally became pregnant," she bitterly told herself, "All that God and my family had required was to watch the baby and keep it safe in my body until the time for delivery." Susan felt so ashamed when she realized, "I can't even do that!" As she anticipated the Christmas gathering, voices began to speak inside of Susan. "You have let your family down. You have failed God."

Susan found a way to pretend that she was sick on Christmas Day and excused herself from joining the rest of the family. She stayed home alone as her husband went over for the customary gathering. Susan remained depressed but refused to talk to anyone about the problem. She tried going back to work but could not concentrate on her responsibilities. She tried attending church but found it too frightening to face a God that she had so disappointed. Her pastor called to see if there was anything the church could do. In the visit, Susan attempted to be brave but suddenly began sobbing uncontrollably. After an extended time of hysterical screams and tears she was still unable to tell her pastor the story: She had failed God.

Pastoral Issues

Self-condemnation easily occurs for some people. Some of these people always see themselves as "bad persons." Some people will always think of themselves as either too thin or too fat, too quiet or too talkative. People such as this are never able to see themselves in an objective manner. Intensive self-evaluation can be very dangerous for such people following a traumatic experience. People who see themselves in a negative manner will often find ways in which they may have brought their trauma upon themselves. They will examine their lives and find ways in which they may have displeased God and, therefore, deserved their trauma. Instead of seeing themselves as victims, they will see themselves as receiving their "just due." In Susan's case, she saw herself as causing her miscarriage. No matter what her physicians may have told her, she could only blame herself. She saw herself to blame for the argument, for the miscarriage, and for disappointing all of Mike's family.

People like Susan create extended and difficult problems for themselves at a time of pregnancy loss. Since a loss such as a miscarriage is so personal, these people will not be comfortable in discussing it with others. Unfortunately, they have a problem that falls between two professions: medical and spiritual. These two professions are likely to face the problem in part rather than as a whole. Susan may be able to discuss some of her feelings of guilt with her pastor but may find it very awkward to go into detail regarding her guilt for not being able to ovulate properly. She may discuss the ovulation problem with her physician, but that person may not be able to understand her feelings of guilt. She is left on her own to put the two professions together and solve the problem from her own ability to see the "big picture." Unfortunately, Susan and others like her often are unable to see a bigger picture. They need the two professions to see beyond each one's specific territory. It would be extremely helpful if Susan's pastor would develop a comfort level in discussing personal health problems with individuals. Often, if pastors are comfortable with such conversation, the people will develop a similar comfort. That level of comfort should not be difficult to achieve, even in the current era when pastors have significant fears of sexual charges. Susan's pastor should feel comfortable in letting her talk about her leg if it were broken. Why should it be asking too much for the pastor to become comfortable in hearing Susan talk about her ovulation?

As Susan developed further manifestations of guilt, she entered into a behavior similar to the account of the first human guilt experience. In Genesis, Chapter 3, Adam and Eve introduce a behavior referred to as "hiding." After eating the fruit, Adam and Eve could not specifically identify what had gone wrong with them but knew that something was not right. They needed to find healing in God. Instead of going to God, they attempted to do the opposite of what they needed: They tried to hide from God. This type of hiding behavior is seen in many who have undergone pregnancy loss, such as Susan and, in the previous account, Toni. While needing to find healing in the ministry of the church, these people, instead, pull away from the church.

Effective ministry requires delicate handling of these "Susans." If confronted too strongly, they will only retreat further behind their walls. Only a patient and compassionate pastoral caregiver will be able to allow Susan to ask for help in facing her guilt. Jenny, in the next case study, will illustrate an even more serious case of "hiding." In both situations, the hiding is very detrimental to healing. The withdrawal from the church by grieving people is a withdrawal from one of the primary settings God uses to give them the grace to experience the nurturing and healing that they need.[4]

Both Toni and Susan present an additional problem of ministry. Churches are often considered as places where families come to celebrate. Those who are not able to celebrate may find the church a difficult place to enter. Religious holidays can intensify these problems. Thanksgiving, Christmas, and Easter are often holidays that focus on the blessings of family life. For someone like Susan, these holidays following a loss are not likely to invoke very much celebration. Instead, these holidays will create a reminder of what will never be in life. Unless the church is aware of people like Susan and the unique needs that they bring with them as they face certain holidays, the church will never understand these people always seem to be absent on those special holidays.

Every church must be aware of the weak points in its ministry. Most churches are not equipped to handle individuals like Susan. While well-intentioned in recognizing and supporting the family unit, many churches will actually reinforce the guilt people like Susan experience. She had no choice in her problems with ovulation, nor would Mike have had a choice if he were the "problem" in having a low sperm count. Yet, these people are often excluded from celebrations on family Sundays, particularly on days such as Mother's Day or Father's Day. Often, they are excluded from the celebrations as if they had defied God's order. Not being a parent may even lead to being treated as lesser persons in many churches. Until churches learn how to celebrate their "Mikes and Susans" they will add to the problems of guilt and "hiding" behavior. Perhaps the simplest solution is to recognize all adult men or women on these days rather than just those who have parented a living child.

While struggling through these family holidays, Mike and Susan may find special pressure to be in church during these family oriented holidays when they are so vulnerable. Just like the setting for Steve and Toni, churches may even add further to the problem by expecting their "Mikes and Susans" to be involved in the workload of putting on family programs. Mike and Susan need to have help in easing up their life schedules as these holidays approach. These events may often bring the grief experience back to these people. Churches need to be supportive to these unique settings.

While we have focused on the needs of Mike and Susan, we have not addressed the needs of the extended family. Should they be held at fault for wanting a male descendent? Are they at fault for celebrating with Susan's announcement of her pregnancy? Further, who will care for their grief in knowing that their family name may forever come to an end?

CASE STUDY THREE: "I HAVE SINNED"

Jenny had difficulties throughout her life. Although she sometimes tried, Jenny never did well in school. Her parents never thought she could be trusted with much. They weren't even the least bit surprised when she was the only one of twelve in her confirmation class to not receive confirmation.

Jenny's parents began to see her as more than just a person who often failed. They began to think of her as a disaster. These expectations were regularly being communicated to Jenny.

By age twenty-one, Jenny began to get good at disaster. She had already experienced the failure of two marriages. She had quit four jobs and had been fired from three others. She had tried two colleges and, predictably, failed at that, or so she claimed. Despite the marriages not working out, she had three children, all with different fathers. She recently had another relationship fail. The man walked out on her, leaving her pregnant for the fourth time in as many years.

Jenny went through an otherwise normal pregnancy only to have the baby born dead. The doctors explained that the umbilical cord had wrapped around the baby's neck and had choked the oxygen supply during delivery.

While all sorts of failure seemed to come natural to Jenny, and she found herself able to even joke about it, the failure of her baby to survive delivery left her with traumatic impact. She no longer seemed able to care about anything. Her sister, Cindy, agreed to take the other three children "for awhile." Neither Cindy nor her husband wished to do so but consented under pressure from the children's grandparents.

Even with the ease of having the tasks of motherhood taken from her, Jenny did not respond to life as she had in the past. She no longer appeared able to cope with any difficulty, no matter how small. When she made an attempt on her life, she was admitted for psychiatric care. Two weeks later she was back in her apartment. Cindy's pastor, Reverend White, was asked to visit Jenny to see if he could provide any help. After a brief but less-than-helpful contact with Jenny's psychiatrist, Reverend White set up a time to visit with Jenny.

Reverend White was surprised to discover that Jenny was extremely willing to talk about herself. She revealed a life that was loaded with self-destructive behavior. Most of her failures stemmed from actions that she performed knowing that the consequences would be destructive. Reverend White was even more surprised to hear Jenny speak of her relationship with God. Jenny saw herself as someone cursed by God. She could quote endless verses of scripture to indicate why God would want to curse her. However, in her mind, until now she alone was the victim of her failure. Now, her baby had become the victim of her failure. Jenny believed that God had taken her baby's life as a payment for her sins.

Jenny had strong support for her view. She could argue that she was not a fit mother for the child. If any mother deserved to lose a baby, she felt she did. Having been in church for many years, she had become acquainted with Biblical accounts. She discovered Biblical cause for her stillbirth. She showed Reverend White the passage of II Samuel 12:14 where David's infant son was killed as a result of David's adultery. "Because of my unfaithfulness in keeping my marriage vows," Jenny claimed, "God has taken my child as well."

While Jenny seemed to have strong support for her disfavor with God, Reverend White somehow found the argument too simplistic to believe. "After all," he thought, "how many families would have had pregnancy loss if it were the direct result of sin?" More than he could imagine. Also, didn't Paul see himself as the "chief of sinners." Why did God allow him to live? Yet, the logic seemed to weigh heavily in favor of Jenny's argument. What should Reverend White tell her?

Pastoral Issues

Jenny presents a difficult setting for ministry. She does not see herself as worthy of God. She is so convincing that even her caring pastor found it difficult to debate her logic.

Jenny represents many contemporary people. In spite of the fears of sexually transmitted diseases, a large number of people are participating in premarital and extramarital sexual relationships. Many carry significant guilt over these relationships. Many of these same people may not fit into the church culture and, unlike Jenny, do not receive large doses of Christian education. Like Jenny, they may spend much of their life in church and still not come into contact with the doctrine of grace. They feel bad about themselves and assume that God does as well. They may engage in self-destructive behaviors and then not be surprised when bad results occur.

How does Reverend White present Jenny with an experience in God's grace? How does he help her change a life of negative self imagery? She had already been baptized. Would another baptism help? She claimed to have been converted many times before. Would another time be of help? What about her understanding of scripture? Should the passage of David and Bathsheba be weighed against the passages of Ezekiel 18:4, 13, 17, 20, which indicate another message? Will introducing such passages only confuse Jenny and imply that there may be contradictions in scripture?

Jenny poses a difficulty problem in pastoral care because she starts with a poor concept of God and builds her life upon that concept. She expects her life to have a lack of blessing (failure) and creates her own expectations. Should Reverend White confront her with a sense of responsibility for her life choices or should he present her with an experience of grace?

Even being with someone like Jenny is risky for Reverend White. After all, Jenny did not dress with the modesty that others in town do when visiting a pastor. Reverend White is a single man who is worried about rumors. Jenny will need extended care. What might the church people think if Jenny comes back to the office on a regular basis? Is Jenny too great a risk for such ministry?

People who fail a lot are not likely to become productive church members anyway. Based on recent financial reports, Reverend White's church needs tithing members. Jenny is not likely to reward Reverend White and his church with anything material if she were to become a regular attender. Should Reverend White be spending his time with better prospects?

CASE STUDY FOUR:
"AT LEAST YOU HAVE EACH OTHER"

Jim and Pat have had a successful relationship with each other. They first met while in college. It was "love at first sight." Pat felt that she had finally met the man who could understand her needs. They were married two years later.

During the time of courting, Jim noticed how dependent Pat was upon her father for his approval. Even as a young adult, Pat still loved to sit on her father's lap. Jim learned a great deal by watching Pat receive affection from her dad. Jim did his best to meet her needs by giving her plenty of attention and affection. Whenever she was discouraged, Jim would make sure she was cheered with plenty of kind words and romance. It was all so easy for him because Pat clearly displayed her emotions and made it obvious when Jim was meeting her needs.

When Pat discovered that she was pregnant, she was not very happy at first. She wondered how Jim would respond. She hoped that he wouldn't be unhappy. After all, they were not well-off financially and Jim was now thinking about graduate school. As soon as Jim revealed his excitement at her news, Pat felt relieved and soon shared in the joy herself.

While Pat's sister had difficulty during her pregnancy the previous year, Pat experienced no such problems. Both Jim and Pat worked through the transition problems together. When Pat wondered if she no longer looked attractive because "she was so big," Jim would give her a hug and assure Pat that she was "as pretty as ever." Pat appreciated Jim's sensitivity and Jim felt secure in knowing how well he met Pat's needs.

When the baby finally came, two weeks late, Jim was more than ready to celebrate. He waited a bit for Pat to come out of the delivery room before he began to call friends and family to tell of the good news. However, Jim couldn't help but notice a concerned look upon the obstetrician as he stepped out of the delivery area. The obstetrician pulled Jim over and said, "You need to stay with Pat; we are not getting good results on your baby's heartbeat."

As Pat was taken to her hospital room, Jim stayed close by her side. As the alarming news was being given to Pat, Jim gave her a big hug smiled, and said, "Just wait and see; our baby will pull through." Pat smiled back.

The wait for further medical reports seemed to take an eternity. However, during the wait, Jim, as usual, knew the right words and the right ways to provide touches to maintain Pat's outward optimism. For just a short while it appeared that Pat was beginning to cry. However, Jim gave her a big hug and kiss. The tears left Pat's eyes as she returned Jim's kiss. Pat and Jim realized how important it was that they have each other during the crisis time.

Unfortunately, the baby did not "pull through." Several days later the baby's heart stopped. Efforts to resuscitate proved futile. Both Jim and Pat were in complete shock as they watched the events take place. To Jim's surprise, Pat shrugged her shoulders as she looked at Jim and said, "Well, now you can plan on your graduate work."

A few hours later the reality began to set in. As Pat was waiting for her discharge from the hospital, she began to hear the cry of other babies in the nursery. She saw expectant moms walking the hospital hallways. She saw the look of joy on parents who anticipated their baby's birth. Suddenly, her grief came upon her like the attack of a mugger. Pat's entire face convulsed as she led out a scream that echoed down the hallways. Jim tried to grab her shoulders only to watch her limp body fall upon the floor. Jim helped the nurses get Pat back on her bed. Pat's screaming and sobbing continued. Watching Pat grieve suddenly brought a grieving experience to Jim. He looked to Pat but realized that she could not help him. She was totally unaware that anyone was in the room. Jim looked to the staff but they were all anxiously leaving the room, closing the door so that others would not be disturbed. Eventually a chaplain came. She stayed for a time but was paged into the emergency room. She promised to come back in "just a minute." However, before the chaplain's return, the floor nurse finished the reports for Pat's release. Pat and Jim suddenly found themselves getting into their car, not sure whether or not to go home or simply sit in the hospital parking lot. Over and over again, they looked at each other. Then they would look at the floor. After what seemed to both like an eternity, Jim started the car and headed home. During the entire distance—some two hours—no words were spoken. While both liked the same music and usually listened to their favorite station while they drove, neither Pat nor Jim bothered to break the silence by turning on the radio.

Once home, Jim helped Pat get situated on their bed. Somehow, the bed seemed different from the place that they had known. It seemed like such a cold place; not at all like the place where their baby was conceived just a short time ago. As Jim left the room, he gave Pat a limp hug, closed the door to the nursery across the hall, and went into the garage to work on his antique car, a project that had pretty much been on hold since the pregnancy began.

"Things just weren't the same," Jim somehow thought, two days later. "I keep giving Pat those same hugs that I used to give her, but they don't feel the same. She doesn't seem to notice I'm even touching her half the time."

Jim's sense of uneasiness soon turned to guilt. He now was free to begin graduate work. But somehow, even though she didn't say so, Jim felt like Pat resented that he was looking forward to the education. Jim tried to reason with Pat. He explained, "With the education we could be financially better prepared for the next child. This situation could only get better with the loss." It all made sense to Jim. He even hoped that Pat would agree with him one day as he shared his sense of relief that the baby didn't live. "The next baby would come at such a better time for everything," he attempted to explain. With that, Pat let out a scream similar to her scream at the hospital. However, when Jim tried to help her to a chair, Pat pushed Jim away. To pretend he didn't notice the rejection, Jim escaped into the garage to work on his car.

Rejection set the tone for the next several months. For Jim, each evening had the same routine. Jim came home from work, ate a bit, and headed for the garage. In a few weeks, Pat went back to work and developed her own routine. After dinner, she always headed into a back room to watch television or simply stare into space.

Jim was the first to become unhappy with the change in their relationship. He often tried to hug Pat in the manner that formerly seemed to be very helpful. He pretended to not feel the rejection when it didn't seem to cheer her. He even tried being more romantic. However, it became such a task that he stopped. One night he thought she was trying to wake him up with the beginning of a sexual relationship, but he found it hard to respond and they both fell back to sleep. The struggle seemed so unfair to Jim. Before, romance had come so easily for him and Pat. He wondered, "What are we doing wrong?"

Soon, Jim's patience began to grow thin. At work, he heard other men talking about their sex lives. Previously, Jim would even lower himself and enter into the conversation to brag about his times with Pat. However, now Jim found himself quickly walking away and pretending he didn't hear them.

One day Jim came home determined to make things just like they used to be. He presented Pat with a dozen roses and gave her his most romantic embrace. However, Pat could return none of his feelings. Hours earlier she had been at the grocery store and had met an old college friend whose baby was born the same week as their baby. In seeing this baby, Susan could only grieve her loss. Instead of being romantic, Pat could only turn away from Jim and begin sobbing.

Jim took it all very personally. He threatened Pat that if she wasn't going to be passionate again he could find plenty others who would. He really didn't mean to say it that harshly, but it all came out so fast. With that, Pat took the roses and shoved them at Jim. The thorns painfully went through his shirt into his chest. Jim stared at the roses on the floor and the blood on his shirt. He began to apologize. However, he noticed that Pat had returned to her back room and was again looking out into space.

Jim couldn't believe that Pat was the same woman with whom he had fallen in love. As he looked at her, he felt so repulsed by her appearance. He began to remember the old days when they were so in love. Why couldn't he bring those days back?

Next Sunday, Jim went to church. He had been missing church quite frequently since Pat became pregnant. That was so unlike him. After service, he shook hands with the pastor and explained that things weren't very good. However, the pastor patted him on the back and said, "Well, at least you have each other." With that the pastor began greeting the person behind Jim.

Pastoral Issues

The church often implies specific roles for husbands and wives. Traditionally, the husband has been expected to materially provide for the family. With the miscarriage, Jim would be able to fulfill that role in a more effective manner. Was Jim wrong in being relieved that the next baby could come at a better time?

What should Jim have done in trying to cheer Pat? Was that his role? Is there something else he could have done? Can he be blamed for trying to help her along?

What is the role of the wife in a Christian marriage? Is she always expected to meet the sexual needs of her husband? How soon after a traumatic loss such as her's should she be expected to be her cheerful and sexual self again?

What is the role of the griever? Is it normal to grieve a baby for several months when the mother hardly even saw the baby? The physician warned Pat that the baby was likely to have trouble. With all the warning, shouldn't Pat have avoided becoming attached to the baby? By failing to heed the warning, in some way did she deserve her problems?

Pat and Jim took conflicting roles in grief. Pat tried to "feel" her way through grief. She seemed unconcerned that her need to experience grief was contrary to Jim's need to "consent" and go on. He was back to his old self the same day that Pat came home from the hospital. His approach to grief lead to a much more productive lifestyle than did Pat's approach. After all, he was working on a hobby, getting ready for school, and was back to supporting the family immediately after the loss. Since his approach to grief was so productive, wouldn't it, therefore, be much superior to Pat's approach?

Why did the pastor think that his statement, "At least you have each other," would be helpful to Jim? Why did it not provide much help to Jim? What could have been more helpful?

Why would touch and sexuality become different to Jim and Pat after the loss of their baby? Can a marriage be expected to survive this change? What could Jim and Pat do about it?

CASE STUDY FIVE: "GOD FAILED ME"

Even good friends often referred to Sharon and Bob as "health nuts." This was not without reason. Sharon and Bob were always concerned about things that might affect their health. Neither one ever touched alcohol, tobacco, or any nonprescription drugs. In fact, neither one would even take an aspirin unless they were in extreme pain. Both seemed almost compulsive about their health. They watched their diets for fats, cholesterol, sodium, and anything that might be harmful to their bodies. They religiously took special care of their bodies with daily rigorous exercise. Both practiced safe sex and were virgins up to their wedding night.

Sharon's sister, Alice, was just the opposite. She had a sexual life that embarrassed her entire family. In fact, Sharon was embarrassed with nearly everything that Alice did. Sharon had tried to convert Alice to a healthier lifestyle many times, but all without success. When Alice announced that she and her current "significant other" were expecting a baby, Sharon became much more aggressive in pushing her values upon Alice. Sharon insisted that Alice stop using the illegal chemicals and severely restrict her use of alcohol and tobacco while she was pregnant. Alice seemed to agree with Sharon. In fact, at first Alice was a model mother-to-be. But the changes were too drastic for her and soon Alice was back to her old habits. In spite of all the warnings from Sharon, Alice was consuming both legal and illegal drugs on a regular basis. This led to a sharp fight one night as Sharon preached a "fire and brimstone" message to

Alice. Alice responded in a nasty tone and demanded that Sharon leave her apartment forever. Sharon left in anger that night, not feeling bad that she was unable to tell her sister the good news that she, too, was pregnant and shared a due date just four months after that of her sister.

In time, both began to feel a bit childish for the fight. Neither felt comfortable with making the first contact. However, months later Alice had a reason to initiate a call. She had just delivered her baby and couldn't help but tell Sharon the good news. Her baby was born in good health but, because of some chemical abuses, needed some special care. Alice even asked Sharon if her church friends would pray for her baby, "just in case." Sharon couldn't believe the change in Alice, who never before appeared to have any interest in religion.

With great expectation, Sharon brought her minister to see Alice and the baby at the hospital. Neither Sharon nor her minister, Pastor Heather, were at all judgmental about Alice's lifestyle. At the end of the visit, Pastor Heather even offered a baptism for Alice's baby. However, Alice wasn't up to that much religion and politely declined. Sharon eventually reported to her church that Alice still needed their prayers as the baby was fine but that Alice had a new partner and was planning to have a child with him.

With Alice back to her ways, Sharon decided to concentrate on the last weeks of her own pregnancy. Everything appeared to be fine until the expected week of delivery. During her last prenatal examination, the obstetrician suddenly had an unusual look upon her face. It concerned Sharon but she acted like she didn't notice. Suddenly, a whole host of hospital staff burst into her closet-sized clinical room. They began looking, poking, and eventually hooked some strange machines onto her tummy. She tried to find out what was going on but the staff seemed too busy to respond. Just as fast as they all came in, they all left. A sudden sense of fear came over Sharon as she prayed silently.

About twenty minutes later her obstetrician and a few others entered. Sharon knew something was up. Her worst fears were realized when they told her that they could no longer find a heartbeat on her baby.

Several days later Sharon gave birth to her stillborn baby. The delivery was extremely painful, even for all the emotional preparations Sharon had made. Sharon's husband, Bob, and Pastor Heather were there with her during the entire time, providing wonderful support.

As Sharon returned to her room, things seemed to make no sense at all. Pastor Heather asked if there was anything that she could do for either of them. Bob had no special needs. However, Sharon asked Pastor Heather if she would baptize their baby before he was taken for a funeral. Sadly, Pastor Heather felt it necessary to refuse on both requests. "The church cannot baptize the dead," Pastor explained, "and a funeral for a stillborn baby is not in keeping with the church tradition either."

With that, the normally calm Sharon exploded. Suddenly, she threw her water glass at Pastor Heather and cursed loudly, both at her and at God. "You would baptize my sinful sister's baby but won't do anything for mine," she yelled in her hurt. "Besides," Sharon shouted even louder in words normally far from her vocabulary, "what kind of a God do you represent anyway? My sister lives like an absolute heathen, takes poor care of herself, and is rewarded with a baby. I take good care of myself, am faithful to God, and get this. What good is any of this religion if God can't even watch over a baby?"

Pastor Heather tried to provide answers that she had learned in a counseling course in seminary, but each answer just made Sharon more angry. Meanwhile, an apologetic Bob was helping Pastor Heather with a towel. While not waiting to let her clothes dry, Pastor Heather dismissed herself without offering a prayer.

Eventually things smoothed over between Pastor Heather and Sharon. However, Sharon just never seemed to care much for religion anymore. Even though Bob remained a loyal and active member, Sharon stopped attending all religious functions. Her lifestyle began to show unusual changes away from her normal concerns for personal health. Bob tried to understand, but found himself confused. Whenever Bob tried to get an explanation for her changes Sharon would only say, "If God rewards sinners like my sister, why should I go to the effort to live like a saint?"

Pastoral Issues

Have you noticed that God may not always reward peoples' lives in a just manner? Why should that be? In Mark 11:22-25, Jesus promises that our prayers will be answered, "Whatever you ask for in prayer, believe that you have received it, and it will be yours" (New International Version [NIV]). Did God fail or did the prayers for Bob and Sharon's baby fail? Who lacked the faith: Bob, Sharon, or Pastor Heather? Would the baby have survived if Sharon would have prayed with even more faith?

In Psalm 139, we read that God's creation of babies begins while they are yet in the womb. The Psalmist writes, "You knit me together in my mother's womb" (NIV). This indicates that God designs babies before they are born. Can one expect that God cares enough for these babies to form each one properly? Why didn't Sharon's baby have that kind of care?

Was it wrong for Sharon to be angry at God? Was it wrong to be angry at Pastor Heather? Did Pastor Heather need to respond to Sharon's anger? What will God do to Sharon for being so angry? Would not expressing her anger have been better or would it have lead to worse problems?

Could Pastor Heather have provided anything like a baptism or a funeral for the baby? Are there any rituals that she could have used? Does the death of the person end the church's ministry to that person? What about the needs of the surviving family to have a ministry to the baby's body?

Why did God answer the prayer for Alice's baby but deny the prayer for Sharon's baby? Shouldn't God reward Sharon rather than Alice? What would one say to Sharon? What would one say to Alice?

CASE STUDY SIX: JUSTIFYING GOD

Steve and Sandy had been active in their church. They were "team teaching" the Adult Bible Study on the Book of Romans each Tuesday night during Sandy's pregnancy. One of Steve's favorite verses had been Romans 8:28, "And we know that in all things God works for the good of those who love him, who have been called according to his purpose" (NIV). Even though Sandy was having difficulty during her pregnancy, she did not worry because she knew, "God would work it for good." After a long and difficult delivery, Sandy finally delivered a baby boy. Both Steve and Sandy were so delighted to have their life expectations met in a baby. They had been hoping for a boy and had even picked out his name: Justin.

However, within an hour after his birth, Justin suddenly died. The abruptness of the loss overwhelmed Steve and Sandy. A loss such as this was not what her Bible study taught her to expect. This was far from working out toward good.

The physician promised an autopsy, which might give them some answers. For Steve and Sandy, that seemed so helpful in trying to find some "good" in their loss. During the six weeks while waiting for the autopsy report, both felt more and more confused by the loss. They waited expectantly for the autopsy report date, hoping that it would give them some sense of meaning to their loss. Unfortunately, their physician could give them little information. They were told that their baby had immature organs and was not able to sustain life. With that, the physician shared his sympathy and excused himself.

Steve and Sandy found no meaning for the loss in the autopsy report. Certainly there was nothing that might indicate some form of "good" in the loss. Their other quests for meaning in the loss resulted in the same lack of answers. All these events seemed so uncharacteristic of the God that they thought they knew. None of it seemed to have any connection to the promise of Romans 8:28.

Steve and Sandy turned to their friends at church. They began to ask others to pray that they might find their answers. Soon, various members of their church tried to help them by giving answers that they thought would help ease Steve and Sandy in their loss. Some indicated that God was glorified by the way that Steve and Sandy gave testimony to their God during the memorial service. Others told them that Justin must have been a special child and that God wanted their baby in heaven so he could be loved sooner than other children. Another suggested that Justin would have grown up to give them nothing but heartache. God took Justin to avoid any such pain to Steve and Sandy.

While these answers met the needs of friends, Steve and Sandy found little meaning to the helpful suggestions. They did not think that their child needed to die for God to be glorified. They felt bitter that God would penalize their special child by denying him life. While Justin may have caused them pain, Steve and Sandy were insulted that God didn't think that they could handle the problems that Justin might bring to them.

More answers continually were being given to Steve and Sandy. One friend suggested that it was because Steve and Sandy were not in church often during the pregnancy. That person thought that the death was God's way of "bringing them back into the fold." This suggestion infuriated Steve and Sandy in that they didn't think it fair that they couldn't miss church a little bit without suffering such a terrible punishment. They wondered, "Didn't God understand how sick Sandy was those Sundays that she missed church? Why did Justin have to die for their sin? Wasn't Christ's death enough?"

Others indicated that the loss was just something that they would "get over" in time. After all, "they were still young and could have another." Another impressed that, "They should be grateful that God allowed this to happen so early in their lives when they had plenty of time to replace Justin."

Steve and Sandy felt very confused as they continued their search. Finally, the months went by and people slowly stopped giving them answers. In fact, people appeared to simply lose interest in the topic. Steve and Sandy were still very much interested in the topic and focused upon it every week. About six months after the loss, a member of their Bible study confronted Steve and Sandy in a rather nasty tone. She told them, "If you don't get off this Justin issue, I and others here will stop coming to this study. We all have to get on with our lives and the issues that we face. You need to move on as well. Besides, if you can't accept these problems in life, what would you do if you had a real problem, like the death of a spouse?"

Neither Steve nor Sandy could understand why they felt so hurt by the comment. Sandy remained a leader in the Bible study and willingly moved to other topics. Steve chose to stop leading the Bible study and eventually dropped out completely.

Pastoral Issues

Those who tried to counsel Steve and Sandy had several deficits. Unfortunately, they had no awareness of their deficits. None of the friends in the Bible study were aware that they had not suffered from Justin's death at a level anywhere near the level that Steve and Sandy felt. None could provide counsel because they did not understand the issues involved. Perhaps that was why they could "get over it" so quickly and Steve and Sandy could not. That would be why the individual in the Bible study couldn't see Steve and Sandy's loss as "a real problem." That would be why they could not compare this loss to a loss of spouse. Is it possible that Steve and Sandy may have found Justin's death more painful than the loss of a spouse? Perhaps Steve and Sandy could not really imagine the loss of a spouse. Would Justin's death be more painful than an imaginary loss? Would Steve and Sandy be wise to use their own timetable rather than follow another's schedule for grief?

Hopes for logical answers seemed to end with the autopsy report. This end is a familiar disappointment for many grievers of pregnancy loss. Unlike deaths involving older children and adults, autopsies for unborn and newborn deaths seldom give clear information on causes for death. With so little information with which to work, those who counsel grievers will err in trying to respond with logic. Such a logical approach will be seem appropriate. Those who have not experienced the depth of the grief, such as Steve and Sandy's friends, will understand logic. However, Steve and Sandy are in grief. Grief is not logical. All of the friends tried to respond with their logic, and this had a predictable result. What would have been more helpful for Steve and Sandy?

Perhaps the most comprehensive question would be, "Why does there have to be an answer?" Romans 8:28 does not indicate that people will always understand how good will come out of all situations but, somehow, God will make it happen. If God gave Steve and Sandy a "reason," would they be able to understand it or would their finite reasoning lead them into further confusion? Was there any possibility of success in their quest for a reason?

Deaths such as these push our faith to the limits. Some people find themselves needing to "justify God" by giving an excuse for things that do not make sense. It becomes easy to find all sorts of "reasons" for God's actions. However, such justification never seems to accomplish much. Does God really need us to "justify" divine actions?

CASE STUDY SEVEN: SOLO GRIEF

A pastor asked me to visit Cathy, a member of his church. He indicated that she had experienced a miscarriage and was having difficulty with her grief. As I visited with her, her husband walked in wishing to join us in telling of the experience of loss. We talked for hours. Even though the loss was over a year ago, it seemed as if they spoke of something that had just occurred that very day. They gave a very complete chronology without, it seemed, sparing any painful details.

After an extended conversation, Cathy asked me if I would like to hear her poems that she had written for her baby. I acknowledged my appreciation for such a privilege. She poured her husband and I each a large cup of coffee and then poured her soul before us in her writings. As she went from poem to poem we found ourselves laughing, crying, grieving, and celebrating–sometimes together, sometimes not. Finally, Cathy indicated that she couldn't read any-more. I looked at the clock. We had been talking of their grief experience for some six hours. It was well past midnight. As I thanked them for their time I began to wonder, "where was her grieving problem?" I asked her, "Are you able to function enough to get by since the loss?" Cathy responded in a most unusual man-ner: "Up until now, I don't think that I have. However, knowing that another person cares about us makes life so much more manageable."

I began to wonder what I actually did that night. Her pastor called me later and told me that I had worked a miracle. It soon dawned upon me what I had done. I had validated her loss. In another later visit, I discovered that she and her husband had tried to share their experiences with others but could find no one interested. She even tried sharing her poems, but no one seemed interested in hearing them. Eventually, she resigned herself to the fact that she and her husband were alone in the loss.

In later visits Cathy's husband, Ron, began to be more involved. He began to ask questions. "What happened to our baby?" was often a topic of concern. "I hear that our baby was simply sent down a garbage disposal at the hospital," he would add, "I sure don't feel good about that. Couldn't the hospital let us provide our baby with a decent burial? I've asked a number of people at the hospital that very question. They don't seem to understand why I feel like I do."

More concerns eventually came from Ron. He wondered if he would see his baby again. "How will I know him/her if we meet in heaven? Will individuals like our child be a baby or an adult?" I had no clear answers for Ron but helped him discover peace in a lack of answers with a faith in trusting God.

Pastoral Issues

Why would it appear that Cathy is not handling her grief very well? What was her need? Why wasn't this need being met?

Why would Ron and Cathy's church not have been receptive to hearing these accounts and poems? Can otherwise good Christians sometimes lack sensitivity? How many churches would be willing to give Ron and Cathy an audience?

Why would Ron be uncomfortable in not having cared for the body of his baby? Why would a hospital not understand his feelings? What could have been done for this body to give it more dignity?

Isn't the idea of people, whether alone or as a couple, "going solo" in grief an expansion of the initial tragedy? What should the church do to keep this from occurring? What can you do?

NOTES

1. L.G. Peppers and R.J. Knapp. *Motherhood and Mourning*. New York: Praeger Publishers, 1980, p. 66.

2. Kohn, I. and P. Moffitt. *A Silent Sorrow*. New York: Delacorte Press Bantam Doubleday Dell Publishing Group, Inc., 1992, p. 77.

3. Davis, D.L., PhD. *Empty Cradle, Broken Heart*. Golden, CO: Fulcrum Publishing, 1991, p. 56.

4. Mayfield, J.L. *Discovering Grace in Grief*. Nashville: Upper Room Books, 1994, p. 69.

Chapter 3

Philosophy of Pregnancy Loss Ministry

UNDERSTANDING YOURSELF IN MINISTRY

All people who are in a ministry setting will bring a series of theological values with them into their service. Much of this theology is not made visible to most people involved in receiving ministry. Sometimes, this theology is not even visible to the ministers themselves. They may have a theology that guides them, but they are often not aware of the values or definitions that comprise their theology. Instead, this becomes a hidden agenda. Neither the persons nor their co-workers can fully explain the values that are behind their ministry–values that are quite often inconsistently applied–nor do they even know why they arrive at their theological destinations.

When such blind spots occur, the ministry will become lost without any sense of direction. Unless the ministry team is comprised of members who are a perfect clone of each other, they will not be able to coordinate themselves because they are not able to coordinate values. Even the individuals within the team will find themselves unable to coordinate their individual ministries as they will continually have unexamined, contrasting values.

Examples of this can be seen in many ways. In some instances individuals who do not know their values will cover their vagueness by describing themselves with general terms such as having a "counsel-based approach" or a "Bible-based approach." Yet these persons will be very vague when pressed for more details. They will be vague because they are not aware of their own values toward loss, suffering, or grieving.

This ignorance is most unfortunate and sometimes dangerous. Unless a self-evaluation takes place, the ministering person will be providing counseling sessions and expressing totally unexamined values. This becomes counterproductive at best. If the caregiver does not know his or her own theology of ministry he or she is capable of erratic use of various different values. This is not a setting for effective ministry.

For this reason, people in ministry need to have an established value system in which they can operate. It is not the purpose of this writing to impose values as much as to help individuals speed the process of understanding and developing these values. In this brief section, the reader will find various containers in which their values can be identified and brought out for application.

DEFINITIONS AND THEORIES OF LOSS

It is important to know oneself as a person in ministry because personal values can often be transferred upon people to whom we counsel. However, having an understanding of self also demands that there also be a definition of terms. For example, each support worker's personal expectations for "normal grieving" will be used as a tool for measuring grief resolution. The support person may encourage further professional counseling for those who are not in the expected "normal" range. It becomes extremely important for each support person to develop a "normal" that is in harmony with a mainstream normal versus an imagery that is too often literally "plucked from the air." A definition of "normal range" must be discovered and evaluated for each one who is involved in grief ministry. A wonderful practice session can be obtained by using this and other definitions with the pastoral issues of Chapter 2 in developing a measurable style of ministry. Such styles can be evaluated by the individual caregiver or with other caregivers so that a common language can be developed.

Two contrasting methods of facing grief also need to be understood. While there are many different approaches that one can take involving grief, two opposite values can be found between those who will take a "consenting" approach against those who will tend toward an "experiencing" approach. The former tend to become stoic in facing life experiences while the latter will explore personal feelings from their grief experiences.

Consenters

Consenters are those able to move beyond their experiences without much introspection. These people tend to expect both good and bad from life and never take either extreme very seriously. When a loss occurs, such as pregnancy loss, they are able to move beyond the tragedy onto "other things" with relative ease. They do not necessarily accept the loss but instead learn how to consent to it and move on with their life. While consent may seem similar to denial and is often mistaken for it, there are differences. Denial avoids the problem. Consent adapts to the problem.

The positive side to the consenting approach is demonstrated in its practical values. These people do not need much time off from work for their bereavement. In extremes, they may be fully functional in all their responsibilities the same day of their loss.

Many societal values will encourage this approach, especially in pregnancy loss. Since most people will have little bonding experience with the baby, they will have no feelings of grief in the death. They may consider the grief of the parents or other family members as "strange" or "inappropriate" for "just a baby." Society can be very rewarding for those grievers who will reflect consenting values. Society will reinforce these persons' lack of grief.

Rewards can be very high to those who adapt consenter values. Often, job promotions or pay increases will be based on virtues such as the lack of time missed for personal reasons. This virtue will be expressed in terms of "job loyalty" or a "positive work ethic." Usually, employers will speak very loudly when these values are either supported or violated by workers.

A negative side to consenter values begins with the dangerous practice of "capping emotions" not altogether different from a practice of those in denial. Such attempts to cap emotions can be like attempting to cap a volcano. It will not stop the force but instead make the eventual eruption even more explosive than if left to make a natural release.

Persons who are allowed to slow themselves in matters such as taking time off from responsibilities to do their grief work will often be less likely to have emotional problems further along in life. Those who return to normal life too quickly may also discover that they have to come back to the problems and work through experiences that would have been better dealt with at the time of loss when support systems are more available. In the long run, this "capping" of emotions may cause people to be even less effective in their work life than those whom they criticize by being "stuck in their grief."

Another negative side to consenting is that the person may be very productive for less than productive reasons. The grieving consenters may spend endless amounts of time and money changing light switches in the house, replacing all sorts of parts to the car, and endless other hours being busy and "productive" so that they do not have to experience their grief. They may even be so busy that they change jobs, move to a new home, and plan a career change. In the process of doing these things, they are not mentally prepared for the decisions and end up much worse off than they were originally. People in grief often will make life changes that are not well considered. Many such persons have made decisions that have caused financial, emotional, or other devastation simply because it seemed appropriate at the time. Such busy activity may provide quick remedy for the grief but later be of greater problem. Meanwhile, the consenting griever's partner is alone because the consenter is too busy to provide emotional support. Societal voices can be very silent while all this is happening.

Experiencers

Experiencers are the opposite extreme of "consenters." While no griever will ever be at either polarity, most people will find themselves leaning slightly toward one side or another. "Experiencers" are the persons who are very reflective about the events of life and their personal involvement in these events. These people will be very reflective about the events in their pregnancy loss. The reflective times will create significant episodes of grief.

Experiencers will have the ability to work through their grief and eventually move on to other things. However, they need time to accomplish that task. They will spend time in grief and generally grow from the loss. They may even be able to create meaning in the experience. Experiencers will have many accomplishments from their approach even though they may not have the tangible results of the consenters.

Experiencers can have problems in that they may withdraw from life and can become negligent to their obligations. During their times of grief they may become completely undependable. If there are not people to carry their load for a time, they will create one difficulty after another. This can have a terrible rippling effect upon their lives. Failure to function at their employment can lead to a loss of job and thus to loss of their home and consequently to all sorts of other troubles.

A further difficulty occurs when the grieving person is matched with another who has a differing grief style. In American culture, one often discovers that the mother in pregnancy loss will be the experiencer and the husband or father will be a consenter. While this should not be assumed the pattern, it will occur in the vast majority of situations. In the first case study of the previous chapter, this pattern was seen in Steve and Toni. The lack of grief congruency between the two partners can lead to many relational problems, even greater than displayed by Steve and Toni or even as serious as those of Pat and Jim.

Ministry workers naturally tend to support the side of which they personally would take in a loss. It is important that the ministry worker not side with one or the other but enter into an appreciation for the approach of each griever. If ministry workers have not discovered their personal grief preference, they will unknowingly take sides.

The next three terms, Theories 1-3, are not necessarily as contrasting as were "consenters" and "experiencers." These terms demonstrate various approaches to suffering and loss. The terms will be helpful in understanding the different ways in which many people approach pregnancy (or any other) loss. They all occur when the person is able to identify some element of meaning to loss. This meaning may or may not be immediately visible to the person. Some situations may combine more than one or all three. Theory 4, "Suffering and Loss Have No Meaning," will be an opposite to Theories 1 through 3 and Theory 5.

Theory 1: Suffering and Loss Are Times of Testing

Those who support this pattern will see a God who is judgmental—who wants to know our "true colors." The Book of Job gives significant support to this pattern. Job was tested by Satan to determine his real faithfulness. In spite of all that happened, Job was commended by God for remaining true through his testing period. In the New Testament, many references are found for this endurance. Hebrews 11 speaks strongly in this manner. Jude and other apocalyptic authors, including the writer of Revelation, also emphasize this theme.

We read in II Timothy 2:3-5:

> Endure hardship with us like a good soldier of Christ Jesus. No one serving as a soldier gets involved in civilian affairs–he wants to please his commanding officer. Similarly, if anyone competes as an athlete, he does not receive the victor's crown unless he competes according to the rules. (NIV)*

In Matthew 10:22 we read Jesus' words:

> He who stands firm to the end shall be saved. (NIV)

In James 1:12:

> Blessed is the man who perseveres under trial, because when he has stood the test, he will receive the crown of life that God has promised to those who love him. (NIV)

In James 5:11:

> As you know, we consider blessed those who have persevered. (NIV)

This theme has been strongly expressed throughout the history of the church. Many of the early church martyrs were motivated to not renounce their faith so that they could be "faithful through their test." One such clear message of this value was seen in the Donetist Schism of the fourth century, involving questions about those who

---

*Scripture taken from the Holy Bible, New International Version. Copyright 1973, 1978, 1984 by International Bible Society. "NIV" and "New International Version" are trademarks registered in the United States Patent and Trademark office by International Bible Society.

had not been faithful. The church faced the question: "Was it acceptable to accept such 'failures' back into the fellowship?" These "failures" were on trial for not persevering "to the end." While the Donetist Schism has come and gone, the questions have remained with the church.

The church has numbers of people who feel that the Christian life is a struggle and that the highest virtue is to "pass the test." They may also see judgment from God for those who do not pass this life test. The account of Job is very relevant in our time because many still see suffering as a sign of God's judgment. These people fill the role of Job's comforters even today. In pregnancy loss, these comforters will "help" the bereaved family find reasons why they may have failed the test. These comforters will not allow grievers to express their feelings of doubt or question for fear that in such expression, "they may not pass the test." This can create significant problems for those who need to express themselves and ask questions that might reflect doubt.

The strong side of those who see the suffering of pregnancy loss as a "test" is in giving meaning to a very meaningless experience. After a loss, the family is generally left with doubts about themselves, God, and the future. The "testing" approach often gives a very simple but usually adequate meaning to tie all of the meaninglessness together into a purpose. The grieving person can realize that this is a temporary experience that has a clear reward at the end. They can go through their daily sufferings with the assurance that there is "light at the end of the tunnel."

The approach of seeing pregnancy loss as a test also unites the person with countless other persons who share a common experience. People suffering from pregnancy loss can find others who have undergone significant testings in their lives. They can share their experiences with these persons who can provide excellent support during this current trying experience.

The testing approach to suffering also allows the person to avoid feelings of judgment. "After all," the person will reason, "everyone, good or bad, is tested in some manner." The person undergoing suffering can see that their misfortune has not come as a result of God's displeasure upon themselves. "If others have undergone this testing," they will think, "I need not feel bad that this testing has also come to me."

Viewing pregnancy loss as a testing also provides the griever with a sense of hope. Since no test lasts forever, those who see pregnancy loss as an experience in undergoing a test will realize that if they remain faithful to the end of the test they will receive the same fate of other faithful. "Hope is just down the road," they think.

The negative side of the testing approach has already been mentioned. Many who are "experiencers" will need to express their doubts. They need to have room to do so without "failing the test." Those who are not allowed to do so will often retreat from the church.

Throughout history many have seen suffering from a testing focus. Clement of Rome, writing perhaps before the end of the first century, saw virtue in "testing" by discovering ways in which the strong persons can help the weak ones:

> In Christ Jesus, then, let his corporate body of ours be likewise maintained intact with each of us giving way to his neighbor in proportion to our spiritual gifts. The strong are not to ignore the weak, and the weak are to respect the strong. Rich men should provide for the poor and the poor should thank God for giving them somebody to supply their wants.[1]

Origen sees meaning in this testing approach as he states in the early third century from his commentary on the passage from I Corinthians 10:13:

> For as the officials of public games do not allow competitors to enter the lists indiscriminately or fortuitously, but after a careful examination, pairing in a most impartial consideration either of size or age, this individual with that . . . so also must we understand the procedure of divine providence, which arranges on the most impartial principles all who come to engage in the struggles of this human life, according to the nature of each individual's power, which is known only to Him who alone beholds the hearts of men.[2]

Luther, in the sixteenth century, added support with his statement:

> It teaches us, not how to avert it by our effort and resistance but patiently to endure it till it wearies and exhausts itself upon us, can do no more, and of its own accord ceases and drops from us in impotence, as the ocean waves dash against the shore, turn back and disappear. Not yielding but perseverance counts in this conflict.[3]

Historically, the belief that God allows times of testing has continually been taught as a source of meaning in times of suffering. It has served well as a source of hope for those to whom the struggle has been long. Contemporary ministers will find this approach helpful to themselves or to grievers as long as the struggling Christians are allowed to have and express emotions and doubts.

Theory 2: Suffering and Loss Are Times of Training

Scripture often indicates that suffering is a necessary process in which we become better people. The author of Hebrews 12:5-13, in quoting Proverbs 3:11 and 12, states:

> And you have forgotten that word of encouragement that addresses you as sons: My son, do not make light of the Lord's discipline, and do not lose heart when he rebukes you, because the Lord disciplines those he loves, and he punishes everyone he accepts as a son. Endure hardship as discipline; God is treating you as sons. For what son is not disciplined by his father? If you are not disciplined (and everyone undergoes discipline), then you are illegitimate children and not true sons. Moreover, we have all had human fathers who disciplined us and we respected them for it. How much more should we submit to the Father of our Spirits and live! Our fathers disciplined us for a little while as they thought best; but God disciplines us for our good that we may share in his holiness. No discipline seems pleasant at the time, but painful. Later on, however, it produces a harvest of righteousness and peace for those who have been trained by it. Therefore, strengthen your feeble arms and weak knees. Make level paths for your feet, so that the lame may not be disabled, but rather healed. (NIV)

The author clearly considers enduring hardships as God's way of making us better people. He even indicates that we should welcome it in knowing what we will gain from the experience. We see this even further in James 1:2-4:

> Consider it pure joy, my brothers, whenever you face trials of many kinds, because you know that the testing of your faith develops perseverence. Perseverence must finish its work so that you may be mature and complete, not lacking anything. (NIV)

Many leaders of Christianity throughout the centuries have proclaimed this approach to suffering. St. Ambrose, in the late fourth century wrote:

> A blessed life can rise up in the midst of pain.[4]

Clement of Alexandria, writing perhaps in the early third century, saw suffering as a means of learning about our sins:

> The suffering the Sodomites endured was a judgment passed on those who sinned, but for those who hear the story, it is education.[5]

Gregory the Great, writing about the year 600, saw suffering as a means of betterment of the soul:

> The stones for building the Temple of God were hammered outside, that they might be set in the building without the sound of hammer. Similarly we are now smitten with scourges outside, that afterwards we may be set into the Temple of God without the stroke of discipline, and that the strokes may now cut away whatever is inordinate in us.[6]

Luther, in the 1500s, responded to suffering with a metaphor:

> It requires the art of believing and being sure that whatever hurts and distresses us does not happen to hurt or harm us but is for our good and profit. We must compare this to the work of a vinedresser who hoes and cultivates his vine.[7]

John Wesley, writing in the 1700s, perhaps merged Theory 1 and 2 to say:

> It is by sufferings that our faith is tried, and, therefore, made more acceptable to God. It is in the day of trouble that we have occasion to say, "Though he slay me, yet will I trust in him. And this is well pleasing to God, that we should own him in the face of danger; in defiance of sorrow, sickness, pain, or death.[8]

There are many positive sides to this approach of suffering as a means of education or training. Those who see suffering as a growing or learning stage have a "completely packaged" meaning to their sufferings. They, like those who see suffering as a test, can find hope in the shortness of the suffering as it needs to exist only for a short time.

There is a point of superiority of the training approach over the testing approach. Those who are tested are often subject to evil powers. For example, Job was placed in the hands of Satan to bring him harm. Those who are being disciplined or are going through a learning process can be completely in the control of God. There is a significant increase in feelings of peace in the latter approach. There is also significantly more freedom in expressing feelings in this approach than against the testing approach. The person who is training feels free to grunt and even whine a bit during the growing process. Those who are being tested feel a need to be more stoic to prove their faithfulness.

The negative side of seeing suffering as a means of growth is very similar to the down side of the testing approach. The package is too simple. Significant questions are not addressed. In pregnancy loss, the family is left with no reason why a child must die so that they can "improve." That does not appear to be the natural order of God. Some may become so angry at their teacher, i.e., God, that they display their emotions by wishing to intentionally fail the training session. Others may just quit on their growth completely.

For the latter reason, it can be helpful to view Satan or other evil powers as the ones who are allowed to bring the sufferings so that God is not the direct author of suffering. This has a down side in that it takes people away from God's immediate presence. However, it can take away the possibility that God would cause evil to come upon an individual.

Theory 3: Suffering and Loss Are Mysteries of God

This has biblical support in such passages as Luke 13:1-5:

> Now there were some present at that time who told Jesus about the Galileans whose blood Pilate had mixed with their sacrifices. Jesus answered, "Do you think that these Galileans were worse sinners than all the other Galileans because they suffered this way? I tell you, no! But unless you repent, you too will all perish. Or those eighteen who died when the tower in Siloam fell on them—do you think they were more guilty than all the others living in Jerusalem? I tell you, no! But unless you repent, you too will all perish. (NIV)

In these passages, Jesus warns people against assuming that they can identify a reason for unexplained tragedy. The point of the passages appears to be that certain bad events "seem to happen no matter what people do." The reader is left with the identity of tragedy in a mysterious form.

This same concept is shared by Jesus in Matthew 5:44-45:

> But I tell you, Love your enemies and pray for those who persecute you, that you may be sons of your Father in heaven. He causes his sun to rise on the evil and the good, and sends rain on the righteous and the unrighteous. (NIV)

This is a significant contrast to Amos 4:7:

> I also withheld rain from you when the harvest was still three months away. I sent rain on one town, but withheld it from another. One field had rain; another had none and dried up. (NIV)

This does not indicate contradiction in scripture as much as contrast in scope. The former text appears to be speaking of a general action of God in relating to humanity while the latter refers to a specific, abnormal action of God. The Matthew text appears to be the one that is most indicative of God's normal working.

All of this indicates that there is a mystery to tragedy and suffering. Perhaps there is a danger in trying to identify for ourselves or another, "Why God allowed something bad to happen." This is further indicated in the Book of Job where the comforters and Job were confronted with their complete inability to understand God and therefore unable to resolve the mystery of suffering.

An approach such as this can be very helpful in ministry to those suffering from any loss, but particularly to those suffering from pregnancy loss. Generally, following a loss, people become very introspective. This can be both good and bad. It is helpful because it allows people to become more aware of their own finitude and to plan their remaining time of life. It is less than helpful in that some people will begin to blame themselves for the loss. A mother who has experienced pregnancy loss may blame herself for either not exercising enough or being too active and therefore, "causing the baby damage." The father can also blame himself for placing too much demand upon the mother while she was pregnant. Most couples who experience a pregnancy are young and not well-off financially. Life demands are increased with the pregnancy. Most couples can find plenty of events that occur with these demands that may have stressed the mother's body and, thereby, caused the pregnancy to have ended in loss. Unfortunately, much of this ends in blame or some form of scapegoating. Blame and scapegoating usually become terribly destructive, and in pregnancy loss, comes at a time when the victims are extremely vulnerable.

In contemporary society (perhaps as in any era) the sexual mores of a society will be much higher than the likelihood of most of societal members to fulfill the mores. This can create all sorts of focus for "reasons of God's judgment." Often the couples will blame themselves for the death because one or the other may have been sexually involved outside of and/or before the marriage. It is not hard to let this lead to terribly destructive introspective analysis.

Instead of placing blame or needing a place for blame, the persons going through grief can be encouraged to accept their finitude as mortals that limit their ability to understand the reasons behind the suffering. The persons going through this loss can focus upon their grief needs and move along in life. They can progress as they are ready without becoming sidetracked on futile attempts to understand that which may ultimately be understandable.

Doctrines describing suffering as a mystery are not new. John Chrystostom, in the late fourth century wrote:

> Some people, out of restless curiosity, want to elaborate idle and irresponsible doctrines which are of no benefit to those who understand them, or else are actually incomprehensible. Others call God to account for his judgements and struggle to measure the great deep . . . For when we struggle to learn things which God himself did not will us to know, we shall never succeed–how can we, against God's will?–and we shall gain nothing but our own peril from the investigation.[9]

Martin Luther, in the sixteenth century, added:

> Would you expect a prince to divulge all his plans and decisions to his people and confide all his policies to his subjects? Should a general reveal, make known, and publish his tactics and strategy in an encampment? That would be some army and business! And yet we fools, in the devil's name, will not believe our God unless He has previously initiated us into the why and the wherefore of His doctrines![10]

There are many recent writers who have provided us with many volumes on this topic. In his classical writing, *The Problem of Pain*, C.S. Lewis challenges Christians to recognize that the ability to experience suffering is a part of the divine image placed upon us at creation. Lewis insists that we cannot have the image of God unless we are willing to accept suffering. To not have the experience of suffering would be to become a lower form of life. Lewis portrays suffering as a mystery we need not avoid but rather accept, just as Christ accepted the cross and was glorified by the acceptance. By his model, Lewis shows how the mystery of suffering can be more than just endured by seeking God's will through the experience.

The practical application of this theory occurs when the caregiver is able to realize that pregnancy loss has come for reasons unknowable to humanity. It can be very soothing for the caregiver to reach this conclusion. In other approaches, such as seeing pregnancy loss as a sign of God's punishment, the pastoral caregiver needs to be superior to the one who suffers loss. Otherwise, the pastoral caregiver is also in God's disfavor. By seeing suffering as a mystery, the counselor does not have to be superior. In so doing, any concerns that the caregiver must somehow be superior to the one who has suffered can be removed, allowing for both the caregiver and the one suffering to meet on the common ground of humanity. This alone can create tremendous ministry. In addition, if those who are suffering from pregnancy loss can be helped from letting themselves fall into the pit of self-blaming, healing experiences from the grief can begin much faster and have more effective results.

Theory 4: Suffering and Loss Have No Meaning

This approach has been popularly expressed by many contemporary grief counselors who encourage the griever to "consent" to the loss as compared to "accept" the loss. After consenting to the loss, the individual is encouraged to move along in life. This approach has roots in Stoicism, in both religious (including Christian) and atheistic forms. Many contemporary counselors and psychologists would follow this approach as would much of popular opinion in Western civilization.

Perhaps the most public illustration of this approach in our time has been the Kennedy family. When John Kennedy's sister developed severe cognitive deficits, the family was able to place her in a distant care facility and move along without much sign of visible grief. When John Kennedy was assassinated in 1963, his widow was able to continue life without showing signs of her grief. Neither the earlier death of brother Joseph Jr. nor the later death of brother Bobby seemed to slow the family from their productive lifestyles. Seldom did we see any members of the Kennedy family displaying any grief or seeking to find a meaning for their tragedies. The next generation of Kennedys have not sought to give the losses any meaning in their individual lives. Overall, the American public has been able to be supportive to the Kennedys in their approach.

The strength of this approach is in the way the griever can see the loss as an event that came from a chaotic natural order that has no meaning. Unlike seeing God as moving in mystery, this approach has no desire to find a God who could (or should) have understood or controlled the events of tragedy. Instead, it emphasizes the sufferer's role as a victim, thereby placing the thrust of ministry wholly upon the individual's healing process.

For example, the couple who suffers from miscarriage loss would be encouraged to not seek any meaning in the loss but, instead, reflect upon their feelings of loss and discover ways in which the death has impacted them. The counselor would then support the sufferers to find ways in which these impacts can be either replaced or moved into a location in which the persons can continue their life function realizing that the event had no more meaning than a tossing of dice by nature.

Some further strong points of this approach are to see the counselor and sufferer on the common ground of humanity as also accomplished by the "mystery" approach. No one is better than another when tragedy strikes. All are common victims of these meaningless experiences.

The major negative side of the theory is that it places the sufferer in a position much more distant from God. The experience of David in the 23rd Psalm presented a God who was nearby and perhaps giving meaning to the experience no matter what happened. For those who see suffering as meaningless, while their God is present, often their God is unable to protect them from evil. It may be argued that the 23rd Psalm does not directly indicate that God will protect them from evil. However, the psalmist would be fearful of evil if he were completely vulnerable to it.

The weakness to this approach can be seen in the contemporary book, *When Bad Things Happen to Good People*. While this book has provided tremendous comfort to many people in our time, it is noteworthy in presenting a God who cannot control creation. The author nearly apologizes for God's inability to keep people from suffering. Such an approach can solve the initial grief problem but then creates feelings of insecurity toward future events in a world "out of control."

Theory 5: Suffering and Loss Are Signs of Punishment and Warning

By specific punishment, this definition indicates that each person may discover a specific and different meaning in a loss as well as find a corporate meaning. It also indicates that there is great purpose in discovering the cause of these punishments and ridding oneself of the cause: i.e., sin. Many Biblical sources support this position. Perhaps the best known comes from the Ten Commandments in Deuteronomy 5:9-10:

> . . . I, the Lord your God, am a jealous God, punishing the children for the sin of the fathers to the third and fourth generation of those who hate me, but showing love to a thousand generations of those who love me and keep my commandments. (NIV)

Another popular passage is found in II Chronicles 7:14:

> . . . if my people, who are called by my name, will humble themselves and pray and seek my face and turn from their wicked ways, then will I hear from heaven and will forgive their sin and will heal their land. (NIV)

A further passage comes as a theme throughout the book of Proverbs as stated in 3:7-10:

> Do not be wise in your own eyes; fear the Lord and shun evil. This will bring health to your body and nourishment to your bones. Honor the Lord with your wealth, with the first fruits of all your crops; then your barns will be filled to overflowing, and your vats will brim over with new wine. (NIV)

In these and other passages found in the Bible, the reader is warned that suffering comes to one who is not in a right relationship with God. Conversely, blessings are for those who are in such a proper relationship. In these passages, one senses that meaning can be found in suffering. According to this approach, if one is suffering it would indicate that somehow the person is outside of God's will. Jesus justifies the use of suffering as a warning in Matthew 5:29ff:

> If your right eye causes you to sin, gouge it out and throw it away. It is better for you to lose one part of your body than for your whole body to be thrown into hell. And if your right hand

causes you to sin, cut it off and throw it away. It is better for you to lose one part of your body than for your whole body to go into hell. (NIV)

In reading these scriptures, it becomes clear that such earthly suffering is lesser than suffering in hell and, therefore, a justifiable means of disciplining us into God's will. According to these scriptures, God is providing humanity a service in allowing certain suffering so that these sufferers will not face eternal punishment.

The eighteenth-century writer John Wesley saw suffering from earthquakes as the result of punishment that might be received in a warning.

God is himself the Author, and sin the moral cause, of earthquakes.[11]

Even though there was much death and destruction from the earthquakes, Wesley saw God as the source. The tragedy, according to Wesley, was justifiable because:

God waits to see what effect his warnings will have upon you. He pauses on the point of executing judgement, and cries, "How shall I give thee up?" . . . He hath no pleasure in the death of him that dieth. He would not bring to pass his strange act, unless your obstinate impenitence compel Him.[12]

Finding cause in a specific person's suffering will, then, be of utmost importance to those holding this view. Pastoral caregivers who hold to this view will want to help the person discover a reason for his or her loss. Failure to do so may result in missing God's direction and even finding oneself in eternal punishment. Grievers who hold to this view will also see an urgency in discovering the cause.

In pregnancy loss, such "causes," real or imagined, are often easily discovered. Grievers' simple efforts of reason can reveal many personal defects in themselves or others. This is often very primitive reasoning and can follow certain "folk resolutions" to any other problem. Perhaps the reason will follow that even though the child is innocent and not deserving death, there are specific people to whom something worse than death may occur. The child, not having sinned, will avoid eternal damnation and have an eternity outside of punishment. Most importantly, according to this logic, so will the person to whom the loss is intended to give meaning. As a result, in eternity, everything will work to God's glory (Romans 8:28).

There are a number of less-than-positive sides to this position. Perhaps the most glaring is that the ways and thoughts of God are considered superior to that of humanity (Isaiah 55:8). It becomes very dangerous for people to cross over that line of mortality in attempting to understand God. The result can be worse than the original problem. For example, a family member can find themselves forever ostracized and riddled with guilt because his or her "straying lifestyle" caused the death of a much wanted baby.

Another negative side comes from scripture. Ezekiel 18 expresses a clear message that God does not generally allow one to die because of the sins of another. Reason and experience will strongly question this position as well. If such meaning could be found in a pregnancy loss, then these losses would only occur to "bad people." On the contrary, this is not the case. Some "very bad people" never experience such losses while some extremely good people do suffer this loss. How does one begin to understand meaning in such a confusing setting? Is it actually possible to understand God in this setting? In spite of all of these dangers, this approach remains a common method of coping, especially for those who are dealing with a pregnancy loss.

These are some of the many positions that a caregiver or a griever may take in pregnancy loss. The caregiver needs to be aware of these positions as it will have significant impact upon the way he or she performs pastoral care. Having awareness of positions will allow the caregiver to have set patterns of effective ministry in place for each particular setting.

NOTES

1. Clement of Rome. To the The Corinthians, secs. 37-38. In *Early Christian Writers: The Apostolic Fathers.* Translated by M. Staniforth. London: Penguin Books, 1968, pp. 42-43; as quoted by T. Oden. *Classical Pastoral Care, Vol. 4.* Grand Rapids, MI: Baker Books, 1987, pp. 77-78.

2. Origen. De Principiis. Book III, Chapter II, Sec. 3. In *Ante-Nicene Fathers*. Edited by A. Roberts and J. Donaldson. Reprint edition, Grand Rapids, MI: Eerdmans, 1979, pp. 330-331; as quoted by T. Oden. *Classical Pastoral Care, Vol. 4.* Grand Rapids, MI: Baker Books, 1987, p. 85.

3. Martin Luther. Exposition on Romans 12:7-16, Second Sunday After Epiphany. In *What Luther Says*. Edited by E. Plass. St. Louis: Concordia, 1959, p. 22; as quoted by T. Oden. *Classical Pastoral Care, Vol. 4.* Grand Rapids, MI: Baker Books, 1987, p. 69.

4. Ambrose. Duties of the Clergy, Book 2. In *A Select Library of the Nicene and Post-Nicene Fathers of the Christian Church*. Edited by H. Wace and P. Schaff. New York: Christian Publishers. Reprint edition., Grand Rapids, MI: Eerdmans, 1982, p. 45; as quoted by T. Oden. *Classical Pastoral Care, Vol. 4.* Grand Rapids, MI: Baker Books, 1987, p. 69.

5. Clement of Alexandria. Christ the Educator, Book II, Chapter 8:43. In *Fathers of the Church*. Edited by R.J. Deferrari, 69 volumes. Washington, DC: Catholic University Press, 1947, Volume 23, p. 235; as quoted by T. Oden. *Classical Pastoral Care, Vol. 4.* Grand Rapids, MI: Baker Books, 1987, p. 69.

6. Gregory the Great. Pastoral Care, Part III, Chapter 12. In *Ancient Christian Writers*. Edited by J. Quasten, J.C. Plumpe, and W. Burghardt, 44 volumes. New York: Paulist Press, 1946-1985, Vol. 11, pp. 123-125; as quoted by T. Oden. *Classical Pastoral Care, Vol. 4.* Grand Rapids, MI: Baker Books, p. 35.

7. Martin Luther. Sermon on the Gospel of St. John, Chapter Fifteen, 1537. *What Luther Says*. Edited by E. Plass, 3 Volumes. St. Louis: Concordia, 1959, Vol. 1, p. 17; as quoted by T. Oden. *Classical Pastoral Care, Vol. 4.* Grand Rapids, MI: Baker Books, 1987, pp. 70-71.

8. Wesley, J. *Wesley's Works, Vol. 6.* Salem, OH: Schmul Publishers, no date, p. 236.

9. Chrystostom. *On The Priesthood.* London: SPCK, 1964, republished by St. Vladimir's Seminary Press, Crestwood, NY, 1977, pp. 118-119; as quoted by Thomas Oden. *Classical Pastoral Care, Vol. 4.* Grand Rapids, MI: Baker Books, 1987, p. 65.

10. Martin Luther. Sermon on the Gospel of St. John, Chapter Six, Volume 23. In *Luther's Works*. Edited by J. Pelikan and H.T. Lehmann. St. Louis: Concordia, 1953, p. 81; as quoted by T. Oden. *Classical Pastoral Care, Vol. 4.* Grand Rapids: Baker Books, 1987, p. 64.

11. Wesley, J., p. 387.

12. Wesley, J., p. 397.

Chapter 4

Understanding the Grief
That Results from a Pregnancy Loss

UNDERSTANDING THAT PREGNANCY LOSS
CREATES A LEGITIMATE GRIEF

In *Nothing to Cry About*, B. Berg tells of her experience with medical personal who could not understand her need to cry after she had experienced a pregnancy loss.[1] She indicates that this lack of sensitivity only served to compound her grief. It also caused her additional problems such as feelings of anger, of being misunderstood, and of worry that she was "abnormal" for feeling such grief. Not until much later did she understand that her grief was "normal" and that her tears were actually necessary for her healing. Unfortunately, she did not understand this until much additional and unnecessary damage was done to her grieving process.

While medical personnel have become more aware of grievers' needs since then, many are still in a state of insensitive ignorance. Many within the ministry team of the faith community may also remain in that state of insensitive ignorance. As a result, rather than abiding by the historic oath, "first do no harm," the church can actually compound the grief of these persons.

A number of studies indicate that the loss of a child is at or near the top of grief stress levels. Most people find it at the level of unspeakable horror. In the tragic bombing of the Oklahoma City Murrah Federal Building in 1995, most of us discovered that the death of children in the day care center of that building made the tragedy unbearable. We had to literally look away from pictures that showed rescue crews pulling childrens' bodies from the rubble. Studies during the recent decades indicate that this inability to view is a normal reaction to the death of children. Studies held by Kübler-Ross, 1975; Schwab et al., 1975; Clayton, 1980; and Osterweis, Solomon, and Green, 1984, all reach the same common conclusion that the loss of a child is too painful for most people to even consider. With all of this evidence, it is not hard to imagine that professionals do not want to leave their state of insensitive ignorance. It is too painful for them to see what the person has "to cry about."

While not wanting to see, many also have not wanted to acknowledge a grief involved for those who could not turn away. In fact, up until recent times, grief from pregnancy loss was often not recognized by any of the "helping professions." Pregnancy loss was equated with "tissue loss." It was assumed that both the physical remains and the grief could be disposed in a pattern similar to tissue loss. This held true across most American institutions. Even institutions such as the Internal Revenue Service still refuse to recognize a birth unless the baby was born alive. Only recently have any of the helping professions seriously been able to approach the possibility that pregnancy loss could be a legitimate cause for grieving.

> In the past the survivors of miscarriage were viewed by society as "illegitimate mourners" (Nichols, 1984). Today we are acknowledging their right to mourn. We now realize that parents begin to bond with their child long before the actual birth.[2]

We need to understand that, in pregnancy loss, there is something to cry about. We need to understand that pregnancy loss affects people in all different types of ways that we, as onlookers, might not expect. We need to hear the mourners express these needs and then minister to the people in an appropriate fashion.

> There has been much discussion in the literature of the child's age at death as a determinant of parental grief. Evidence can be provided supporting claims that it is the loss of the young child, the loss of the adolescent child, or the loss of the adult child that is the most difficult bereavement for the parent to experience. Although researchers may argue about it, the clinical evidence suggests that the question is academic and meaningless to bereaved parents. No matter what the age of their

child, parents have lost their hopes, dreams, expectations, fantasies, and wishes for that child.[3]
It does not appear to make a difference whether one's child is three, thirteen, or thirty if he dies. The emotion in each of us is the same. How could it be that a parent outlives a child?[4]

This should not be terribly difficult to understand. Parents who lose their seventeen-year-old child to an automobile accident grieve deeply for that child. Parents who lose an adult child to cancer feel that loss as well. Parents who lose an elementary child to leukemia also feel grief. That same experience is found in parents who lose a child during pregnancy. We need to see pregnancy loss as a valid loss. To a bereaved parent, the loss can be very real.

This movement will not take us into new or unchartered territory. Instead, it will align us with an historic theology. Traditionally, the church has long supported the position that unborn individuals are human. While the actual definition for the beginning of life has not been consistent, historically the church has not had trouble understanding that unborn children would be grieved like any other person. Tertullian, writing around the early third century, states:

> The embryo, therefore, becomes a human being from the moment when its formation is completed. Subsequently, Moses imposed punishment in kind for one who was guilty of causing an abortion on the ground that the embryo was a rudimentary "human being" exposed to the chances of life and death.[5]

With this, Tertullian begins the doctrine of "traducianism" in which the soul is believed to be transferred from parents to the child. This doctrine would virtually identify the beginning of humanity at conception. This long-supported doctrine of the church provides early precedent for the need of ministry to those who have experienced pregnancy loss.

Actually, the belief that the unborn are full and independent persons is even older than the church. The Old Testament implies in Genesis 25:22 that Jacob and Esau were able to humanly interact while yet unborn. Well before the Common Era began (B.C.), Jewish leaders debated the subject. In John 9:2, we read that Christ declined invitation into the debate with his disciples, which indicates that the discussion had become part of the common of the life of the community. Some, even before that time, believed that the unborn human was fully alive and accountable enough to commit sin while still in the womb.[6] These people would, without a doubt, understand that parents grieve the loss of children through pregnancy. Their historic voices question why we now consider this a new ministry or why we now wonder what there is to cry about?

The issues concerning the beginning of life spark plenty of controversy in our day. While one may not want to get into an issue that will bring oneself so explosively close to the issues of abortion, it cannot be dismissed. This also is not unique to our time. Throughout history, the issue of pregnancy loss often has paralleled abortion issues. Athenagoras, writing in the century before Tertullian defines life beginnings based upon individuals who are tolerant of induced abortions:

> For the same person would not regard the fetus in the womb as a living thing and therefore an object of God's care, and at the same time slay it, once it had come to life.[7]

One historian, writing in summation of historical work of pastoral care, writes:

> . . . we see the pastor historically as involved in all stages of the life cycle: present at the birth of children, concerned with prenatal care of souls . . .[8]

The doctrines that compel the church to become involved in ministry to those experiencing pregnancy loss are not only from early church history, but come in very clear detail regarding expectation of the afterlife for these babies. Augustine, writing in the early fifth century expects that life which is lost in miscarriage (abortion as he terms it) or other forms of pregnancy loss, including birth deformity leading to death, will one day be in the resurrection in complete form:

> . . . but who will dare to deny, though he might dare to affirm, that at the resurrection every defect in the form shall be supplied, and that thus the perfection which time would have

brought shall not be wanting, any more than the blemishes which time did bring shall be present: so that the nature shall neither want anything suitable and in harmony with it that length of days would have added, . . . but that what is not yet complete shall be completed, just as what is injured shall be renewed. . . .

. . . And therefore the following question may be very carefully inquired into and discussed by learned men, though I do not know whether it is in man's power to resolve it: At what time the infant begins to live in the womb: whether life exists in a latent form before it manifests itself in the motions of the living being. To deny that the young who are cut out limb by limb from the womb, lest if they were left there dead the mother should die too, have never been alive, seems too audacious. . . . And if he die, wheresoever death may overtake him, I cannot discover on what principle he can be denied an interest in the resurrection of the dead.

. . . and so other births, which, because they have either a superfluity or defect, or because they are very much deformed, . . . shall at the resurrection be restored to the normal shape . . . [9]

The belief that life in the womb is fully life and therefore worthy of grief upon loss is a belief that the faith communities have long held. Ministry to people who have experienced any of these losses should have been developed long ago. Unfortunately, we are only at the genesis stage of this ministry. It is also unfortunate that the focus of this issue is currently placed wholly on the issue of induced abortion with little emphasis left for support toward those who grieve their lost infants.

Ministry to those suffering from pregnancy loss is not a ministry only for those of the church politically siding with the pro-life position. This is not a political ministry. Instead, this ministry expands beyond either political position and should not be seen transcending either political polarity. Only those insensitive to human feelings would concern themselves wondering whether or not the grieving person feels grief through choice. Grieving is not something that one can politically choose to do. There are no political positions that deny the person the right to choose to see their child as fully human, no matter what the child's age.

That the church has doctrinal precedent to provide ministry has importance to the institution of the church. However, the individual griever will have little interest in this history. They do not need our institutional permission to feel hurt. It is real to them whether or not we "approve" their grief. Our ministry is not in giving our approval for their grief but in responding with human compassion to their loss experience. To do so, we must understand what their grief means to them.

UNDERSTANDING THE IMPACT
OF PREGNANCY LOSS

We are still beginning to understand the impact that grief may have upon an individual's life. Many chemical dependency centers have long noted a parallel between those who undergo a significant loss in their life and a later problem with chemical dependency. Suicide prevention centers are now also noting that parallel.

> Evidence that mourning is a disease is persuasive when static methodologies of research are used. Researchers comparing the health of mourners with non-mourners find mourners vulnerable to both illness and premature death. As early as 1944, for example, Erich Lindemann found that mourners are at high risk levels for seven deadly diseases: myocardial infarct (the so-called heart attack), cancers of the gastrointestinal tract, hypertension (high blood pressure), neurodermatitis (chronic itching and eruptions of the skin, particularly in areas of heavy perspiration and in the webbing of the fingers and toes), rheumatoid arthritis, diabetes, and thyrotoxicosis (thyroid malfunction, mostly seen in women). Recent studies have confirmed Lindemann's early work.[10]

This list indicates just some of the physical impact that may occur from grief. Medical science is still beginning to understanding the fullness that grief can impact upon the human body. Other areas of life also may be affected by grief. Medical science is drawing parallels between unresolved grief and an entire assortment of personal problems. These same problems can occur in unresolved grief that comes from pregnancy loss.

The infliction of these parallels with grief are not inevitable if the grieving individual is able to find means for resolution to their grief. Support is crucial for finding such resolution. Providing such support should be the task of local groups such as churches and other faith communities.

Support begins with understanding. Those in ministry need to understand the many ways in which pregnancy loss can have impact upon the individual. The following pages will highlight some of this impact. The effects of grief may be found in many ways depending upon the individual. It may be found upon the person only; upon relationships, which will be subdivided into (1) partner, (2) current children, (3) later children, and (4) grandparents.

Impact of loss can occur on many different fronts. No two grievers will experience their loss in the same manner. It is crucial that the grievers neither be assigned grief impact nor denied grief impact. The grievers should be free to indicate their areas of difficulty and their approaches toward healing.

A Child as an Extension of Oneself

Numbers of studies indicate that people experience the role of being a parent in many different ways. Expectations may be very different even between parents of a common child. Some may identify their child as an extension of themselves. These expectations identify the child as one who will carry on the name, tradition, lifestyle, and even identity of the parent. Personal possessions will be passed along to these extensions. This can explain why many parents are willing to perform all manner of life-threatening acts to keep their child alive. These parents are able to protect their child without regard for self because they see themselves preserved in the child.

The loss of a child who is an extension of oneself is more than an amputation of a body part or a loss of tissue. We all expect that our body will one day grow old and will eventually die. Those who see their children as an extension of themselves literally create an eternal extension of themselves. In II Samuel 7:16ff, King David is promised to have such an eternal extension of himself upon the throne. Following this proclamation we read of David's great delight. He is in awe of the possibility. This level of excitement is often duplicated among those who experience the extension of themselves in a parental relationship. They realize that a part of themselves will carry on into eternity. While the parent cannot comprehend eternity, the parent will comprehend the joy of the mere possibility.

The extension of self should not be considered as a "bad" or "self-centered" extension. Throughout scripture, God has blessed this extension, and throughout the centuries, the church has celebrated it. The need for this extension is a natural need and is experienced by many. It is a very "holy" experience in that the person must first recognize their own mortality and separation from an eternal God.

For this reason, the grief of pregnancy loss has great spiritual impact. Some may consider the act of denying such grief as a sign of "great faith" or "spirituality." It is not. It does not help the cause of God when someone goes on after pregnancy loss as if nothing was lost. Further, it does not help the spiritual status of the griever when the caregiver encourages such denial. Instead, the griever may discover great spiritual benefit from his or her grief. As much as we would like to turn away and not see that anything important was lost, the parent will often force us to see. That same parent will focus anger upon the person who denies him or her that experience.

A Child as an Image of Hope

It is no coincidence that we connect the term "birth" with the term "hope." The two terms have clear similarities. The expected birth of a child comes with great hopes. The birth of Christ was heralded by angels and prophets as a moment of hope for the people. Throughout time, the birth of children has been celebrated with high levels of hope.

Perhaps the most telling indication of the parallel between terms "birth" and "hope" is in a sign found in many nurseries across the country, which states, "A baby is God's way of expressing hope for our world." This popular slogan indicates that such hope is not individual, but a symbol of a hope that is even greater than humanity.

When these expectations are suddenly removed in an event such as pregnancy loss, the individuals involved will sense a loss of hope. It may seem as if a thief has come and taken their greatest symbol of hope from them. The people involved will express all of the emotional responses appropriate for such a loss. This emotional bouquet may include both comparing and contrasting emotions all occurring at once.

Once lost, hope is not easily regained. Studies involving earthquake victims indicate that the trauma that comes from a loss of hope can last for years after the loss. In these studies, victims of earthquakes had their trust of the earth's stability suddenly betrayed. Such people would not readily allow themselves to "trust the earth" again. These feelings of betrayal can last a lifetime and be expressed in many ways, such as nightmares, a fear of heights, a fear of either open or enclosed places, and an extreme panic at any type of vibration upon their body. Such expressions of fear can continually be expressed many decades after the traumatic event has passed.

When birth "betrays" people's hopes, one can expect similar signs of fears. Those involved in grief may find themselves completely paralyzed with fear at the thought of future children. Existing children may find themselves unexplainably "smothered" with protection from family members who are unwilling to trust the world to not harm these children. A whole series of protective devices can be placed upon these children. Because this is such a serious problem, a section later in this book will be devoted to the issue.

A Child as an Image of Success

In a study carried out by Benedek, 1970, parents were identified by children as being of a status near "omnipotent."[11] Parents will often feel comfortable in that status even though they are completely aware of its falsehood. Parents seem to enjoy those moments of having a child look to them with all the respect due to immortals. Even though children will quickly outgrow this stage and eventually see parents as everything but omnipotent, the parent will look forward to and later cherish this time and experience. Parents will see this as having "arrived" at a place of special respect.

While children are mentioned in the Bible countless times as a sign of blessing and success, few passages are as familiar as found in Psalm 127:3-5:

> Sons are a heritage from the Lord,
> children a reward from him.
> Like arrows in the hands of a
> warrior
> are sons born in one's youth.
> Blessed is the man
> whose quiver is full of them.
> They will not be put to shame
> when they contend with their
> enemies in the gate.

In many ways, societal influences still reflect children as a sign of blessing. As our world is recognizing problems of overpopulation, children no longer equal the same clear sign of success of times past. However, the societal rewards will never be eliminated so long as having children is the only means for society to continue.

A Child as an Image of Identity

Whenever people are asked to "tell something about themselves" they will usually include information about their career, their mate, and the number of children they have. These are forms of identity. For many people, to not have children would be the same as not having a career or any other form of identity.

This identity process begins very early in life. This is traditionally, but not only, seen in females. Females, especially but not only, will begin playing house and taking care of their "babies" very early in life. They will develop their roles and the expectations of these roles as parents very early. As the childhood years give way to teen and early adult years, these roles and expectations will slowly be modified and begin to take final form. By the age in which the person is old enough to actually create a child, the person will often have very clear ideas of what he or she expects in his or her identity as a parent.

The effects of such identity are often seen in an unusual form of behavior during the time period just before the baby is due. The couple will often go into a "nesting" stage, in which the entire energy of the couple is focused upon the expected child. At this time, much of the long-laid expectations and roles will come into completion in the identity of the individual. This nesting time can last well into the early life of the child. During this time parents will often place nearly their entire life energy into the child. These are often referred to as the "blur years" in that all events other than those surrounding the child are lost in a blur of distant objects upon which one has no focus. Later, these individuals will be unable to identify historical events, books, songs, or movies that were popular during these blur years, while having full recall of such items both before and after the "nesting era."

When this "nesting time" is suddenly removed, there is a loss of identity. Even though the "nesting stage" is barely begun in pregnancy loss, much of the impact will be seen in full form. This suggests that once entered upon, the nesting stage and its identity are complete. There does not appear to be a need for gradual entering into this stage. Those who suffer as victims from pregnancy loss will often find moments of what may appear to outsiders as bizarre behavior as the grievers seek a means to maintain their identity. Some individuals, both male and female, report finding themselves "parenting" all sorts of objects, both alive and inanimate. Some find themselves cradling any object that may appear about the same size as a baby. A rolling pin, a cat, a head of lettuce, or any other item may be employed to fulfill the need. The person may experience a desire to fulfill their identity as a parent upon any such object.

While all of these items may provide a release, it ultimately cannot fulfill the complete identity of "parent" for the individual. The person may even have other children in their life, either current or subsequent to the loss. These children will not fully remove the feeling of incomplete identity as "one part will be continually missing." This loss of identity needs to be understood and become an area of support and ministry.

It should not be assumed that these forms of identity are found only in females. Males may also have these same needs. Males also may play "parent" in early childhood and progress in their roles and expectations like their female counterparts without the visibility in their engagements that their female counterparts may have. It is terribly erroneous to stereotype this identity need as a "girl thing."

> As the mortality statistics indicate, this is no myth or fairy tale–all available evidence suggests that people do indeed die of broken hearts, men as much as women. The misperception that men are not as greatly affected seems to be based on societal expectations that men need to show their grief minimally in order to demonstrate their manliness.[12]

These losses–extension of self, image of hope, image of success, and image of identity–are far from a complete list of all the personal effects that may occur at pregnancy loss. Some may lose an heir, self-respect, ability to be around children, or other relational capabilities. Some may have undergone severe financial loss in the medical expenses and have serious personal impact resulting from these issues. All of these create significant problems impacted upon the individual in their loss.

GRIEF PATTERNS IN GENERAL

This impact of grief can be displayed in many ways. One of the more typical expressions is found in a prolonged depression-like state. It is not unusual for the person to appear to lack personal energy. The person does not actually "lack energy" any more than would one who has just undergone a long distance run. In both cases the person simply has expended his or her energy in another area and is merely trying to restore the supply. Just as the physical run required extensive energy, so the "grief work" can totally devastate the person's energy supply.

Ministry and support for these grievers can often come from a tolerance of the grievers' inability to carry out tasks that previously appeared easy to perform. Further ministry can occur in helping the person carry out their common daily tasks. Some persons, who have been exhausted from their grief work, will fall far behind in housework or other areas of common living. Help can come from very unskilled but caring people. However, this needs to be done in cooperation with the griever to keep it from becoming a further invasion upon their sense of control.

Since grievers lack energy, it is further helpful to allow them freedom to restrict themselves from all but the most crucial of obligations. Unfortunately, most groups do not understand this need when a member of their group is involved in a pregnancy loss. For example, if the baby were born healthy, both mother and father could justifiably qualify for a parental leave from their employment. If a twelve-year-old child dies, both the mother and father could qualify for personal leave. However, in a pregnancy loss, generally, neither mother nor father qualify for any leave other than a "sick leave" for the mother while she "gets over" her hospital stay. This problem exists in most sectors in spite of numerous attempts to change policies. The person who suffers from a normal grief from pregnancy loss must have other reasons to "justify" his or her grief time.

Grief can also be expressed in forms of reorganization of life. The grievers may discover themselves asking serious questions about themselves, about God, about personal values, or about life direction, to name just a few possibilities. Quite often the issues that are raised by the griever will not be supported by the otherwise available resource systems. Unless the grief is recognized as a valid grief by much of the support system, that system will be unavailable for help. For example, the insensitive church system may not understand the individual's need to question the doctrine of Almighty God. However, the "all powerful God theory" will not make a lot of sense when that God appeared so helpless to answer the individual's prayers for the child's life. That church will often dismiss the issue or try to "talk the person out" of asking such painful questions. If that form of persuasion does not work, many a church has been known to use forms of guilt to place serious pressure on the "doubter." This only makes individuals feel "bad" about themselves for asking a question that would likely have been asked by anyone else in the same situation.

GRIEF PATTERNS IN PREGNANCY LOSS

While there are many studies available on grief, most sources involve extremely complex theories on grief patterns that require rather advanced psychological study as a prerequisite. A more simple pattern can provide a foundation for those who lack this prerequisite. It is found in comparing the types of loss to the generational relationship of the griever. The equation is very simple: to lose a parent is to lose your past; to lose a spouse is to lose your present; to lose a child is to lose your future.

By examining this equation, one can begin to understand why loss of children creates a grief unique to other forms of loss. It is not the same as other losses because it affects a different form of our existence. A child represents our future, and the loss of a child equals the loss of our future. Some, within many churches, would minister to those who have had the loss of a child as they would the loss of a parent or spouse. This is inappropriate. To treat the loss of a child like the loss of our present or past would be like putting a body cast on a person suffering from tuberculosis. While a highly effective treatment for bodies with broken bones, casts are not effective for persons with tuberculosis. It is not that one affliction may necessarily be "worse" or more severe than the other, but that they each require different forms of care. So it is with the loss of generations. The loss of a child is different to a griever than the loss of a spouse or a parent.

This is because the loss of a parent is like the loss of our past. We know that our past is not retrievable. We, therefore, expect to lose our parents just as we expect to slowly lose our past. However, losing a spouse or sibling is like losing our present. Losing our present is a bit less traumatic than losing our past in that the present is ever becoming the past. Thus, we are always losing our present. We, therefore, are more likely to expect the loss of our spouse than we would our children, much as we expect our present to leave us.

The loss of our children, who comprise our future, creates an entirely different setting. Individuals who have lost their future will have no direction in life because they have no future into which they may head. Without a future they have no existence. Without a future, everything has lost all meaning.

These are just some of the dilemmas faced by parents who enter grief for their child. Ministry is different from ministry for other losses because the grief is different from other losses. Ministry to those dealing with pregnancy loss requires much more intense ministry because the grief can be much more intense.

> With the death of a child in the family the blow is felt narcissistically as a threat to the sense of our immortality . . . The bereavement for the child is intimately connected with, and related to, the libidinal investments. The child serves as a tie with the traditional past, but also, and perhaps more importantly, with the future and with our sense of immortality. (Schwartz, 1977, p. 196)[13]

By use of the term "libidinal," the author is stating that the griever of children has suffered the loss of core-level experience and may even experience a loss of his or her sense of being a person. Such grief results are found in an extreme among those who have lost a child, unlike those found in other grief experiences. People who lose their past can continue to function in life rather well. They can simply, "begin the process over again." One does not, "begin the process over again" when one has no place to go.

Pregnancy loss contains all of the elements of a lost future. While many may argue whether the loss of one age of child creates more serious grief than does the loss of another age of child, it appears that all child loss has concentrated elements of the loss of future and loss of self. Pregnancy loss compounds grief in that many will not validate the loss but, instead, treat the griever as someone less than deserving of support. The end result is an individual with intense levels of loss who is left on his or her own to find resolution.

All forms of loss lead to some form of separation. This writing will list some of the ways in which pregnancy loss can impact this separation. While this is simple to comprehend, the application of a ministry response becomes an art. The caregiver should recognize and respond to the impact that may come from these separations. For example, in medicine, it would be inadequate to only know that failure of the heart to function leads to separation of the person and the heart. The medical caregiver must adequately respond to that medical failure in order to provide quality care and preserve life. In the same manner, a ministry of quality care must do more than know the impact of pregnancy loss upon the griever. Quality ministry means that we help provide care for the impact that may come from pregnancy loss. It simply is not enough to give the griever a list of ways in which he or she may experience loss.

While some of this impact has already been mentioned, effective caregiving requires that the provider develop an assessment of the areas in which separation has occurred followed with an in-depth knowledge of the impact of the separation.

There are some works already in existence which may be of help. For example, Elisabeth Kübler-Ross has given us a "stages of grief" approach to those undergoing loss. These stages are:

Stage 1	Denial and Isolation
Stage 2	Anger
Stage 3	Bargaining
Stage 4	Depression
Stage 5	Acceptance

Her stages of grief can be helpful to those who wish to understand the dying experience. Others, such as Glen Davidson, have given us phases of mourning to understand the phases of loss. He prefers the term "phases" in that the term correctly identifies the lack of clear borders that might be found in a term such as "stages." These phases are:

Phase 1	Shock and Numbness
Phase 2	Searching and Yearning
Phase 3	Disorganization
Phase 4	Reorganization

While helpful to many, these stages and phases can prove narrow and limiting for the caregiver. The actual movement from one state or phase to another is not readily determinable. There are no clear boundaries between these stages or phases. Very few people will undergo the process in such an organized pattern as these authors suggest. Instead of expecting the grievers to follow the caregiver's predesignated pattern, it will be helpful to allow those undergoing loss or grief to find their own way through the grief journey. For example, some grievers may become angry before they enter denial. Others may never enter a stage of anger. Some mourners never undergo reorganization. In virtually all situations, one will continually find threads from all stages continually working. Do not allow these authors' stages or phases to force a grief process upon the people of your ministry.

It may be most helpful to allow individuals to write their own pattern of loss and grief. Since the grievers are experiencing the loss of a part of themselves, they may experience some of the five stages of death as described by Kübler-Ross. However, they may also exhibit some of the stages of mourning as described by Davidson. Either way, they need the freedom to follow their own pattern. It may be that more than one stage may be occurring at one time. For example, someone in denial may cling strongly to an expectation that God will heal the child. That person is capable of becoming very angry at anyone who would challenge their denial. Even after coming through reorganizational stages, the individual may forever have a strong element of searching and yearning for their lost child.

This is not to render these organizational patterns as useless. However, instead of expecting the grieving person to fit into a prescribed pattern, it may be better to see how that individual has previously patterned his or her reactions to other issues of significant stress. If anger is a significant coping tool for the griever in other stress settings, it will often appear during the grieving stage in an extended manner. It is not that the person is stuck in the stage of anger, but that the person is using anger as a coping mechanism to create progress through the grief. That person will need anger throughout life for that coping skill. The anger will subside in time but it is unlikely that it will never give way to another "stage." Another person may use faith as a means that could be clinically diagnosed as denial. The person may never see the infant who has died as "gone." Instead, the griever may see the separation as a temporary setting until heaven. One should be very hesitant of taking away such a coping device so long as there are no other significant reasons. Perhaps that grieving person is in better touch with reality than is the counselor. Tampering with that denial may not be helpful to the griever. The ancient rule, "first do no harm," must be respected.

GRIEF PATTERNS IN SEPARATION

Separation eventually becomes a reality in all forms of loss, including pregnancy loss. Ministry can lessen the damage from separation by helping put a wall around the flood of separation. It can be done best by allowing the person to identify the ways in which separation may be occurring. Generally, the grieving person will not be able to provide a neat list of separations. The list will come through careful hearing of the griever's sense of loss. Common separations include:

1. The child
2. The expectations of that child
3. Feelings of separation from God and nature
4. Any items listed in "Impact of Pregnancy Loss"
5. Any secondary forms of loss

Research into bereavement has made it clear that the mourning process is complex and the period of mourning lasts far longer than most people expect. In addition, many characteristics of bereavement are often not identified by the general public as being a part of mourning.[14]

The Child

That there is a separation when a pregnancy loss occurs should be obvious. Unfortunately, many sufferers do not see the obvious. Quality ministry does not assume that sufferers can see that they have lost a child. Quite often grievers will not understand any potential for ministry in their loss. Certainly, grievers will have little awareness of ministry options. Unlike other hospital ministries where the impetus should be from patient request, it is helpful to move the impetus to requests from your suggestions. This means that it becomes more acceptable to suggest potential ministries. To avoid intrusive ministry, there needs to be additional emphasis upon allowing the recipient to decline your offers. A simple solution is to ask the recipient twice for every ministry that results from your recommendation.

A number of ministry suggestions/recommendations need to be made to the griever. Most grievers are intimidated by the institutions such as church, hospital, funeral home, etc., and unable to request any special ministries. Even if able to request, the person may not be aware of any options for ministry. In most cases I have experienced, the griever waited, assuming that the institution would initiate the option availabilities. In many such cases, the griever did not understand that they could have been given items of memorial nature. Most such grievers were also unaware that they could still see their baby even though the infant was not alive. For such persons, it would be unfortunate to wait for them to overcome their intimidations. Instead, suggestions need to be provided.

The Expectations of That Child

Expectations that parents may make of children include all events that a child may provide, whether real or imaginary. The expectations may include a desire that the child would have become a one year old, a kindergartner, a high school graduate, and reach other milestones through life. The grievers of pregnancy loss may have an entire bouquet of such grief expectations come upon them all at once. Naming all such expectations at the moment of loss or any other given moment can be terribly overwhelming. It may be helpful to let the griever identify these expectations over a period of time.

These expectations may require an entire lifetime to fully name. The grievers may visualize their child among other young drivers sixteen years after the pregnancy loss and discover a new expectation that is grieved. Eventually, these expectations may multiply in realization of grandchildren and great-grandchildren that will never come to be because of the loss.

Feelings of Separation from God and Nature

Many religious counselors understand that people may experience times of separation from God. The counselor may misunderstand the feelings of the griever. The counselor may assume that the griever is familiar with Matthew 5:4, "Blessed are those who mourn, for they shall be comforted." The naive counselor may assume that the passage means that the griever will automatically "feel comforted by God" as well. It is naive because, in practice, that is not an automatic experience among grievers. Many in grief, as in the earlier case studies of Chapter 2, may feel they are being punished by God or are experiencing a sense of separation. The idea of a child dying may seem terribly unnatural to the one suffering pregnancy loss. The griever may feel abandoned by God and all of natural order. Such feelings of separation can have a horrible impact upon the person, which magnifies the grief experience.

Secondary Forms of Loss

Areas previously listed in this chapter can all lead to a form of separation directly resulting from pregnancy loss. While these areas include core-level personal issues similar to other forms of separation, they can be minimized with effective ministry. Later chapters will identify specific forms of effective ministry.

Grief that is directly related to the loss can be obvious. Ministry can begin immediately as these more obvious needs are identified. However, other needs, or secondary forms of loss, require more identification. These secondary forms of loss that result from a pregnancy loss can include physical illness, relational or financial problems, or any number of problems. For example, many who suffer from a pregnancy loss indicate that there is a loss of "innocence" from the experience. The person no longer can enjoy the assumption that a pregnancy will equal a baby. If subsequent pregnancies occur, the mother may suffer extreme anxiety attacks if the baby in the womb goes through even short periods of inactivity. The person is filled with knowledge that can be classified as "an afflic-tion" for lifelong worries. These worries can lead to constant anxi-ety attacks throughout the remainder of the griever's life.

Other secondary forms of loss may include problems noted in the earlier case studies. Some grievers may find difficulty in attending activities that were a previous norm. For example, some may find themselves unable to attend church, family gatherings, or any place that places babies or children as a format. The counselor may not easily trace these separations to pregnancy loss. It would be an error to miss the connection.

NOTES

1. Berg, B. *Nothing to Cry About*. New York: Seaview Books, 1981, no page number.

2. Rando, Therese A. *Parental Loss of a Child*. Champaign, IL: Research Press Co. 1986, p. 131.

3. Ibid. p. 6. p. 6.

4. Schiff, Harriet Sarnoff. *The Bereaved Parent*. New York: Penguin Publish-ers, 1977, p. 4.

5. Tertullian. On the Soul. Ch. 37, sec. 2. In *Fathers of the Church*. Edited by R.J. Deferrari. 69 Vols. Washington, DC: Catholic University Press, 1947ff. Vol-ume 10, p. 260.

6. Beasley-Murray, George R. *Word Biblical Commentary, Vol. 36, John*. Waco, TX: Word Publishing, 1987, p. 155.

7. Athenagoras. A Plea for the Christians, sec. 35. In *Library of Christian Classics*. Edited by J. Baillie, J.T. McNeill, and H.P. Van Dusen. 26 Volumes. Philadelphia: Westminster Press, 1953-1961, Vol. I, pp. 338-339.

8. Oden, T.C. *Classical Pastoral Care*. Grand Rapids: Baker Book House, 1994, Vol. 4, p. 143.

9. St. Augustine. *The Enchiridion; or On Faith, Hope, and Love*. Translated by J.F. Shaw from Nicene and Post-Nicene Fathers, Series 1, edited by P. Schaff. Peabody, MA: Hendrickson Publishers, Inc. Vol. 3, p. 265.

10. Davidson, G.W. *Understanding Mourning*. Minneapolis: Augsburg Press, 1984, p. 22.

11. Benedek, T. The Family as a Psychologic Field. In *Parenthood: Its Psychology and Psychopathology*, J.B. Anthony and T. Benedek (Eds.). Boston: Little & Brown, 1970.

12. Davidson, p. 18.

13. Rando, p. 10.

14. Davidson, p. 16.

Chapter 5

Understanding How Pregnancy Loss Affects Personal Relationships

PARTNER RELATIONSHIPS: INCONGRUENT GRIEVING

One would assume that a couple undergoing pregnancy loss would find strength in each other. One would assume that the common loss would be a journey that they could travel together. One would also assume that the couple could comfort each other in their mutual loss, be patient with each other, and support each other as they try to return to a normal lifestyle. However, that is not necessarily the case.

Each parent must complete the grief work in his own way. If parents fail to recognize that each of them has personal ways of grieving and of coping with the grief and the implications of the death, they will set themselves up for additional problems.[1]

Anne Morrow Lindbergh, in her book *Dearly Beloved*, said, "Grief can't be shared. Everyone carries it alone, his own burden, his own way."

She was correct. But for a couple to discover this after burying their child can be shattering. After all, in the back of each of their minds, they believed they could lean on each other as they mourned. But you cannot lean on something bent double from its own burden.[2]

A term used by many caregivers to describe the problem of couples in pregnancy loss is "incongruent grieving," as introduced by

Peppers and Knapp in their book *Motherhood and Mourning*. The term "incongruent" initially refers to any differences between the father and the mother in experience regarding the pregnancy and the subsequent loss. The mother's agenda and schedule may be very different or incongruent with the father's agenda and schedule. The incongruence usually follows a pattern such as this: Before a woman becomes pregnant, she will often have higher levels of anticipation for the pregnancy than will the male partner. She will know of her possibilities of conceiving a child. She will have the first indications of pregnancy, which may occur within a week of the conception. Quite often, rather than risk giving out false joy (or false alarms), the mother will keep information of her pregnancy to herself and leave the father unaware of any such possibilities. The mother will have the thoughts of anticipation toward the pregnancy as she goes to the physician for her pregnancy testing. Often, it is not until this point or later that the mother will share any such information of the pregnancy with the father. When the pregnancy has been determined, she alone will experience a number of body changes. Most of these changes are not immediately observable and, therefore, not experienced by the father. While all the changes are taking place, the mother will likely develop strong emotional attachment to the baby. Even while anticipating the possible pregnancy, the mother is generally beginning to prepare for the impact upon her life that the pregnancy may create. In many cases, the father may have little or no awareness of the pregnancy until this point or even may remain unaware until the pregnancy and the mother's attachment to the baby is even more developed. During this time, he has little opportunity to make any attachments to the baby.

When a pregnancy loss occurs, particularly early miscarriage, the father has had little emotional involvement in the baby. With little connection, he experiences minimal separation. His grief may have been overshadowed by his relief that the mother, to whom he has made significant attachment, was not endangered by the miscarriage. If she was in any life risk, the father could actually be in a stage of relief or even joy while the mother is in a state of separation and grief. He will find it much easier to move ahead from the experience and begin life again.

The mother is often not so fortunate. She will have made significant expectations which lead her to significant attachments. Unlike her mate, the pregnancy loss has not put her in a position where she had the fear of losing a partner. Often she will not be aware of her own life risk. The agenda of her male partner will be very alien to her, especially if it includes feelings of relief. She will have an entirely different agenda from that of the father.

Incongruent grieving often moves beyond this initial stage to a level of deeper hurt. The mother, in her grief, will expect to find support from the father. She may become very bitter at her partner for his lack of grief. She may interpret his lack of grief as a lack of compassion for her or the baby she conceived. She will have difficulty in transcending her experience to that of her partner's.

In her hurt, the mother may find herself making accusations about the father that are not quickly forgotten by either. The father may not understand why she cannot "get over it" and make further accusation back. He may become very insensitive to her feelings and push her to return to a normal life. While well-intentioned, it is no different than pushing someone with a broken leg into walking too soon. The result of his push may only create greater damage.

There is a possibility that incongruent grieving may occur in a reverse pattern. For example, the mother who has an image of unpleasantness in her pregnancy may be relieved that the pregnancy has ended. The father may have had high expectations for the pregnancy and feel strong grief at the loss. While not the norm, this type of grief incongruence is also extremely damaging to the relationship. It has possibilities of developing into something even worse. Societal values often tend to be more forgiving to an "insensitive" or "uncaring" father than to an "insensitive" or "uncaring" mother. Society will tend to join in the "blaming" against the mother rather than against the father when accusations of insensitivity are made. When the mother is the greater griever than the father, her destructive comments about the father will tend not to have as great an audience. Society will forgive his lack of concern. However, if the father is the greater griever than the mother, society may support his destructive comments. For example, he may not understand her lack of grief and question her "worthiness" as a woman for her lacking in his sense of grief. Support for his views may come from a number of sources. Churches can give strong and unhelpful support to his accusations. This can become very destructive to the self-esteem of the mother.

Either way, the incongruence will often create a "consenter" and an "experiencer" role between the two partners. The consenter will seem able to move along with life rather well, "consenting" to the loss and often rationalizing away any impact of grief. The experiencer may continue in an opposite pattern. That person will be totally irrational in grief and constantly feel the impact of the loss. That person will often wish to express feelings with others. Consenters do not make good conversationalists for experiencers because the consenter is trying to move past his or her feelings. Consenters and feelers do not peacefully coexist very well in the same household, at least while grieving is occurring.

The support systems may also be incongruent in grief expectations between the father and mother. Traditionally, the father will be expected to be back at work in a short amount of time after the loss. He will not appear noticeably different after the loss. Often the father will discover that conversation at work or at church will focus on everything but the pregnancy loss. He will be strongly rewarded for his rapid return to productivity. While there have been some recent changes in the use of paternity leaves, he will not likely qualify for any such privilege in his pregnancy loss. In the foreseeable future, even if he qualified for the leave, much of general societal mores would at least "frown" upon him taking a paternity leave if there were a pregnancy loss.

The mother would often have a different setting in her support system. When she returned to her place of work or to other gatherings, people would notice a difference. She may appear significantly different after having given birth. People would be more willing to expect her return to be more difficult than they would the return of the father. They would be more tolerant of her parental leave, especially if it were a neonatal loss. If the loss were miscarriage or stillbirth, the support system, unfortunately, would probably not be as helpful. Either way, the mother will find an entirely different support system than will the father.

Incongruent grieving is displayed in the lifestyle of the consenter vs. the lifestyle of the experiencer. Much like what was shown in the

Chapter 2 case study of Steve and Toni, the consenter often will attempt to avoid grief feelings by staying "busy." Consenters can undergo projects of tremendous energy and time consumption that appear to have very little point or reward. In reality, the reward is in the avoidance of the feeling experience.

The experiencer will find ways to aid the feeling process, and this frequently disturbs the consenter. The experiencer may collect memorabilia, which will be placed throughout the home. Experiencers may desire to have baby items with them as they sleep. All these things help the experiencer feel grief and work through the grief, but can cause problems for the consenter.

In even mild settings of partners experiencing incongruent grief, one cannot underestimate the potential for conflict. It is not surprising that many such couples will experience a high risk of separation in a short time after their loss. However, as psychologist Therese Rando pointed out earlier, this conflict is not inevitable. In simplified form, if each member of the couple can avoid trying to force their grief pattern upon the other, the relationship can still function.

Incongruent grieving is best handled with a supportive outsider who is able to interpret the feelings of the one partner to the other. An arbitrator, often a professional therapist, can explain that both the one "experiencing" the loss and the one "consenting" to the loss are responding in a normal way based upon their settings. If patience can be applied, the two will slowly bring their differences to a common understanding. Encouraging both parties to step outside their own perspective and understand the other's perspective can be very helpful.

PARTNER RELATIONSHIPS: SEXUAL DIFFICULTY

As a couple will often have different grieving responses, so they may also have different sexual feelings in response to a pregnancy loss. One, usually the "consenter," may be anxious to return to a full and active sex life, including plans for a "replacement child" which, the person may naively hope, will remove feelings of grief. The "experiencer" will have other connotations toward sexual intercourse. Sex may no longer be regarded as a "fun" activity. It, instead, may be considered an activity of great fear since it is the surest way to enter another pregnancy loss. The womb may be remembered as a place of death, especially in the case of stillbirth. Such an implication will not connote a positive sexual inference and will make the individual holding the implication hesitant toward further sexual experiences.

The ministry model for this type of setting can be found in the care of couples experiencing impotence or "frigidity" problems. It is important that ministry caregivers realize that this usually requires intensive skill that they are probably not prepared to provide. Professionals with competency in this area of therapy need to be employed. Many such professionals are willing to work in cooperation with a church care system so long as confidentiality issues are not violated. Lesser trained caregivers from the church can still provide tremendous ministry through support and understanding.

Another model for ministry can be found in the care of couples who are experiencing problems of infertility. Again, professional competency needs to be employed in serious problems. In these settings, guilt and shame can become serious factors that hinder the relationship. Sexual intercourse, which at one point was considered a time of excitement for the couple, may degrade into a "job with low expectation of fulfillment." Couples who have this experience relate that it is like "spending the entire day working at their employment only to come home and feel like they spent their night returning to more work." This setting does not create positive self-esteem and respect for the partner, all of which are necessary to healthy sexual relationships. A crucial question for the couple is: "Are we only creating a repeat of our loss?" Some couples will find help in discovering that the probable answer is "No." Others will find help in discovering that they cannot go through life worrying about "what might happen." Either way, unless the couple is willing to live with their answer (or lack of answer), the sexual relationship will be seriously impacted in a negative way.

Whether the problem is incongruent grieving or sexual problems, the caregiver should never assume that enough time has lapsed for the problem to be solved. At best, time eases the sharp edge of the pain. However, the impact can continue decades after the loss.

Often, couples are helped by simply being aware that their problems are not unique.

There are many controversial issues that become involved in ministry to couples struggling with sexual problems. In Chapter 2, Case Study Four, Pat and Jim struggled with sexual issues. Somehow the church needs to help such persons identify their sexual roles in the relationship so that couples such as Jim and Pat can work through their times of crisis. As a caregiver, the church needs to help Pat and Jim sort through their roles that, while having been adequate all through their lives, no longer can sustain them during their crisis period. It is too convenient to dismiss our responsibility by placing this task in the hands of professional sex counselors. While their help can be of immeasurable worth in a crisis such as this, many of the issues in sexual difficulty are religious issues. The church's voice needs to be included. It is wrong to assume that a professional counselor alone will be able to do that. This is seen even more clearly in Case Study Two, where an entire family needed Susan to provide them with a male descendant. We, as a Church, have not been clear on this issue. Do we still encourage our modern-day "Hannahs" (I Samuel 1) to see their role primarily as a producer of children or has the issues of overpopulation changed that emphasis? From God's perspective, did Susan have anything of value that she could contribute to her family and world even if she could not provide that male child? As a religious representative, we need to help our present day "Susans," who will never have the answers to their prayers as did Hannah, and their entire family systems discover their means for resolution. This is a religious task from which we cannot dismiss ourselves.

In working with specific situations, the task is twofold. First, it is helpful to challenge the antiquated values that may become less than helpful in the current setting of the persons involved. Second, it is helpful to keep the grieving persons from becoming the battle-ground of our controversies. Grievers have enough in life to drain their energy without becoming the "front" by which the griever's church and the family systems work through these controversies. It may be necessary that the individuals involved simply learn to appreciate each other even though they cannot agree on these sexual roles. That may be all the task that they can handle while in the crisis.

PERSONAL RELATIONSHIPS:
CURRENT CHILDREN

Pregnancy loss can create a series of problems involving children. There are several excellent sources listed in the bibliography regarding study of sibling relationships in pregnancy loss. Keeping communication open among the surviving children is extremely helpful.

Parents experiencing pregnancy loss have a terrible track record of literally smothering surviving children with protection. Since the loss often comes with little explanation or warning, the parent will rightfully react with fear that another tragedy may occur to the remaining children. After a pregnancy loss, parents can often imagine any of the most horrible tragedies occurring to their surviving children. In addition, parents may not readily accept the reality that their tragedy was, overall, unavoidable. Instead, parents will go to incredible lengths to protect any surviving children. Such parents may also have a difficult time in carrying out discipline of surviving children. The parent may rationalize, "Since the child is alive, I can overlook anything." The surviving children will quickly spot this and can rapidly develop behaviors that are out of parental control. If these problems do not begin to solve themselves in time, therapy may be recommended. One hates to see the unresolved problems of the parent develop into problems of the offspring.

Surviving children of pregnancy loss may struggle in seeing their parents going through the difficulties of grief. Seeing their mom "sick in the hospital" may be very traumatic for the children, regardless of their age. Seeing the parent upon whom they looked for strength appear helpless in grief can have significant impact as well. Parents in grief will find that they have severe energy limitations. Children will quickly feel those limitations and need reassurance that the parent/child relationship will be able to adapt without the child becoming completely eliminated in the parental interest.

Surviving children may have a number of contrasting feelings toward their lost sibling. They may have been jealous of the attention the new child was getting while the family was anticipating the birth. They may have been jealous enough to have feelings of joy when the child was not brought home. They may respond with guilt for having such feelings. They may have also been jealous of their deceased sibling regarding the attention focused upon it after the death. That focus comes at a time when the family has little energy to give to their surviving children. Such children are not able to focus upon their own grief when they have these contrasting feelings of jealousy. These contrasting feelings magnify the problems of the sibling grief.

PERSONAL RELATIONSHIPS: SUBSEQUENT CHILDREN

Many parallels can be drawn between problems faced by surviving children of a pregnancy loss and children born subsequent to a pregnancy loss. However, subsequent children bring problems unique to surviving children. One clear uniqueness with subsequent children is an inappropriate desire that they become "replacement children." Societal pressures may encourage the couple to "hurry and have another child." While a few studies on grieving, such as performed by Lynn Videka-Sherman in 1982, will find value in replacement children, most people find that a quick pregnancy after a loss only adds more problems to their grieving and extends the grieving process. Most agree that serious problems can occur if the next child comes "too early."

In simplest terms, it is difficult to say, "Hello" and say, "Goodbye" at the same time. Pregnancy loss requires that parents quickly do both. The child has barely come into the lives of the family only to require the family to find ways to release the child. Another child being born shortly after the pregnancy loss only muddies the problem. The "Hello" to the lost child can blur into the "Hello" with the subsequent child. At that point the lines between the two children lose clarity. A subsequent child then can become an object of the expectations given toward the previous child who has died. The subsequent child also becomes the object of loss as the "Good-bye" gets mixed with the wrong "Hello."

PERSONAL RELATIONSHIPS: GRANDPARENTS

Grandparents of a pregnancy loss tend to be the forgotten grief sufferers. They bring special needs that are seldom noticed. Medical personnel seldom are able to meet any of their needs. The church, at least, must be aware of their grief so that ministry can be provided.

Grandparents are victims of a double pain. They have lost a grandchild and also see their children suffer. In adding to their grief, they will remember years past when they could hug their children or kiss their scrapes or bruises and the hurts would go away. Grandparents will often have feelings described as "paralyzing" by the reality that this grief has the exact opposite effect. They can do nothing to help their children. No matter what they do or say, the grief remains very acute. Adding to the problem, many grandparents would like to rush in to provide and receive mutual care with their child only to find that there is a spouse that must come first in their child's attention. They may even add an additional hurt if the loss leads them to relive their own pregnancy loss experience from earlier years.

Because of confidentiality laws, grandparents will be the last of the immediate family to be included in the releasing of information by the caring professionals. Physicians will provide information to the parents and surviving children. Physicians seldom have time for questions or needs of grandparents. Grandparents will be left by such professionals to hurt on their own. Even with their needs, grandparents will often be expected to provide support for their grieving children.

Special needs can add to the already complex problem. If there is any level of strain to relationships with their children, the grandparents can find themselves completely outside of the care circle. In earlier eras, grandparents had a bit easier setting since their children were most likely married. In our contemporary era, particularly if the couple is not married, the paternal grandparents may have no rights and no welcome. At this point the hurt may have compounded to such a height that the grandparents simply cannot bear the suffering and literally remove themselves from the setting. This creates a whole new series of family problems.

NOTES

1. Rando, T.A. *Parental Loss of a Child.* Champaign, IL: Research Press, 1986, p. 28.
2. Schiff, H.S. *The Bereaved Parent.* New York: Penguin Books, 1977, p. 58.

Chapter 6

Understanding How Pregnancy Loss Affects Societal Relationships

ORGANIZATIONS

Organizations, no matter how virtuous, tend to focus upon their own self-preservation rather than on the needs of the people involved in their work. All organizations will, at least subliminally, encourage the griever to set aside personal distractions so that their focus can be placed upon the organization. Organizations will not be supportive to the individual displaying needs of extended grief, as this will remove the person from a position of effective service to the organization.

Persons sensing grief in their pregnancy loss experience, or any loss for that matter, will have to remove themselves from the mores of most organizations of which they affiliate in order to experience their grief. The necessity of this detachment can cause further relational problems with the organization. For example, an employer that refuses to allow the employee time for a desired funeral when a pregnancy loss occurs will find that employee becoming insensitive to the needs of the organization. Later, the organization may suffer lack of effectiveness when that employee no longer is interested in making "extra efforts" as before when there are special needs in the organization.

As much as we religious leaders would like to deny it, religious organizations can also be more of the problem than the solution. Much like the church in the first case study of Chapter 2, we may view the members of our faith community as essential for our support rather than people to whom the organization is designed to support.

This insensitivity has an even stronger attraction for churches than other organizations. Churches will see themselves as having important "ends" that can justify their "means" of insensitivity. As Toni's church ignored her grief needs and instead focused upon her failing to care for children in beginning the Vacation Bible School, so any church can focus away from the needs of the person in grief. This is because the church often views itself as serving an important purpose. Quite often it can be justified by making the institution synonymous with God. The church can mandate the pastoral staff toward those ends, as was the case for Toni's pastor. Such mandates can be so extreme that needs of people such as Toni do not appear of concern to any of the leadership.

Such high purpose of serving God may justify a church to push its personnel in all sorts of insensitive manners. Unless we of the faith community realize this, we too, may alienate our people when they need our support. In turn, they will seldom appreciate the insensitivity. Instead, they will return the utilitarian relationship back to the church. A very dehumanizing downward spiral can begin at this point.

The problem and solution is bigger than the immediate issues presented by a pregnancy loss. A pregnancy loss merely magnifies the already existing problem within such churches. The sensitive church must constantly monitor its ministry to be sure that its emphasis is toward people rather than toward itself. If not, the emphasis will become utilitarian toward both staff and people to whom ministry is provided. The church will have no ministry to people suffering from loss of any kind because it will have no ministry except to itself.

FRIENDSHIPS

Pregnancy loss can put tremendous strains upon friendships. Consider, for example, this case setting: Two young women have been best friends since high school. After college graduation they both get married and keep close contact even though they somewhat go their own ways with family and career issues. However, like other events that have happened and of which they have shared together, they discover that both of them are expecting a baby during the same month. Once again they are constantly together and share their daily experiences each night over the telephone. Suddenly, one experiences a pregnancy loss. The other does not know how to respond. Since she thinks that her pregnancy can only remind her friend of what she has lost, she decides not to make further contacts. She decides not to visit her grieving friend until she is past the immediacy of her loss and then only by a telephone contact. The two soon discover that they no longer have much to talk about. Both feel the strain in the relationship. They try talking again some days later but neither can interpret the other's distancing, and the two suddenly stop seeing each other. When the other delivers a healthy baby, the mom who experienced pregnancy loss finds herself unable to come to see her friend's baby. Soon, the friendship comes to a sudden end because of the inability to share important personal experiences. This account is shared over and over between friends when one of them experiences a pregnancy loss. Some people who go through pregnancy loss indicate that this example understates the dramatic manner in which their friendships change. They state that their old friends simply were not supportive. With little energy to waste they choose to spend their remaining efforts seeking new relationships that could be more helpful to them. These friendships may not be long-term relationships but still are helpful in that they are intended to help through an immediate need. Often, however, a whole new level of friendship may be developed.

These abrupt changes in friendships can be very turbulent in faith communities, especially the smaller ones where one such change can upset an entire social structure. A caregiver will often hear the friends of one who has experienced pregnancy loss saying things such as, "She just isn't the friend she used to be." That may be either a sign that the person is becoming a loner and might need more support or that the person is merely changing friends. It is an opportunity to counsel the friend on ways to truly "be a friend." It will open the door for those friends to work through issues in their own lives as well. The worst case response is to encourage the griever to remain in the old relationships because it may be upsetting to the structure of the church.

Chapter 7

Ministries at a Pregnancy Loss

There are many ministries that a church can carry out which can be very helpful to those in the grieving process following a pregnancy loss. A number of them will be listed in this chapter. This is not considered an exhaustive list nor is it a list that, when carried out, will guarantee effective ministry. It is best to allow the grieving persons to confirm whether or not these ministries meet their needs. They may indicate ministry options that are not on the list. The grievers need to be the final judge of whether or not the use of a ministry would be effective in their setting.

SPIRITUALITY AND PREGNANCY LOSS

There are no quick formulas for spiritual recovery from grief. This is because it is impossible to predict how an individual will respond to a loss. In a given grief situation, any of a number of results may occur. For example, one individual may go through a loss and feel that God's near presence was the only support that helped him or her through the difficult times. Another may go through the same loss, sometimes even the partner in the same loss, and respond that he or she felt totally abandoned by God. Some may go through the loss and become closer to God. Some may go through the loss and become more distant from God. The result appears to have little connection to whether or not the person had a close relationship to God before the loss.

With this much incongruence, giving of care will directly depend upon the griever's indication of need. Some will request to have the church reach out and help them. They may even be offended that the church did not come and help without being asked. Others will be offended by having help offered to them. While most churches follow a general rule to minister and support people in grief, it is a myth to assume that certain people may not recover from grief if left alone.

There are other myths involving spirituality in grieving. It is a myth that the church needs to talk people out of any moments of doubt regarding their belief in God. This is not easy for those in ministry because it is not easy to hear people question their relationship with God. This is especially true if it will also challenge, in some form, the listener's relationship with God. However, there are a number of biblical examples that give the griever room to express doubt. For example, during his suffering, Job was not wrong for feeling separated from God. Job was not wrong for doubting that God would give him physical and emotional healing. Job appears to expect that God will heal him through death. In error, Job's comforters try to take his doubts away.

Perhaps an even clearer image is seen in Christ on the cross. As He shouts, "My God, my God, why have you forsaken me?" (Matthew 27:46), Jesus doubts that he will get relief while on the cross. He expresses the terrible separation from God that he feels while upon the cross.

In many churches, the ministry team would try to talk Job and Jesus out of their feelings. Perhaps they would want Jesus to be more positive about his setting. Perhaps they would want Jesus to have more faith. Either way, the result of those settings would not have been quality pastoral care. In the same way, we too, need not feel compelled to talk people out of their doubts. If we try to do so, instead of providing quality care, the door of opportunity to support these individuals will rapidly close.

Many churches might commit another error of attempting to create feelings of separation in people whose grief is healing at an accelerated rate. Such caregivers may have wanted to convince Stephen, as he was being stoned in Acts 7:56, that he was in a stage of denial. These caregivers would want Stephen to recognize and name his fears and have a clear vision of the things that death would remove from him. Fortunately for Stephen, he was allowed to die in dignity and with a sense of victory without such "ministry."

Instead of following these myths, caregivers need to allow grievers to develop their spiritual path through difficult territory. Paths through difficult terrain are slow and tedious to traverse. Quality pastoral care will help the grievers travel without dictating the direction or speed of progress.

The terrain of grief may fit into a series of common grief issues raised by those going through pregnancy loss. They may be described in a series of needs. Ministry should include a means of providing for these needs. It cannot be predicted if some, all, or any of these spiritual needs will be present in any given setting.

SPIRITUAL NEEDS AT PREGNANCY LOSS

A Need To Be Joined with Another Who Has Experienced a Similar Loss

Experience shows that people who have shared a similar loss can provide wonderful support for each other. This is especially true regarding pregnancy loss. Grievers can find significant help in knowing that their experiences are neither bizarre nor wrong. Churches usually have a number of persons among their membership who have undergone pregnancy loss. These people can provide exceptional support for those who have recently experienced a pregnancy loss. Quite often these people naturally find each other within a congregation. They can provide ministry to the newly bereaved simply by letting them know that they are not alone in their grief. These people may even provide a ministry merely by their presence. However, if a church will have a reasonably trained group of people who can provide this level of ministry, they can be much more effective in meeting this need.

A Need To Be Reunited with the Lost Child

This is a spiritual need resulting from a loss of future. Basic questions that come from this need include: Will my child be a baby in heaven? Will my child be in a special place like limbo? How can I know that I will be in heaven when I die? It may include other questions such as issues of "soul sleep" verses "immediate access" into heaven for the dead. These questions may make an otherwise spiritually apathetic individual into one with significant spiritual insight. Although this requires tedious work, the caregiver needs to allow the grievers time to ask these questions. It is wise for the caregiver to be slow in giving answers. If the caregiver is patient, he or she will see significant growth in the bereaved who reach their own conclusions. In many situations both caregivers and grievers have reported wonderful times of growth from the insight that these questions can raise.

These questions open the door to issues that have been of major controversy throughout history. Some caregivers or other well-meaning church friends will attempt to impress their opinions upon the griever. Unfortunately, this is usually a waste of effort in that the griever will often develop his or her own opinion in a short matter of time. Others will provide "information overkill" to those who are taking on issues of controversy. This, too, is a mistake. The person who asks these questions during grief will generally suffer from a lack of energy. Another characteristic of grief is that it may temporarily take away the griever's attention span. People who lack energy and attention span are not benefitted by large amounts of information that will confuse them and require large amounts of energy in order to find reconciliation. The caregiver should help grievers digest all of the raw data into pieces that are easy to understand and helpful to the spiritual walk through grief. The griever is usually seeking to find comfort in the reality, "I will go to him, but he will not return to me" (II Samuel 12:23).

A Need to Find New Hope

Grievers often lose their sense of hope. The world that they trusted has betrayed them by taking something precious from them. Grievers will find difficulty in regaining their trust in life. Caregivers err in dismissing this lack of trust. It is very real to the griever and, if not resolved, will cause very serious reactions in life. Such reactions may lead to unusual panic episodes, especially regarding the safety of surviving or future children. If the problem persists, professional therapy may be needed. Either way, support is essential. Otherwise, panic episodes will only further damage the person's well-being and be detrimental to the targeted children.

Other needs may occur, generally with less frequency than the ones previously listed. These are a need to find a meaning for the loss and a need to find a reason for the loss.

A Need to Find a Meaning for the Loss

Some people will seek a connection between their pregnancy loss experience and a meaning that is greater than the loss itself. The meaning may be found in a memorial tribute for the child. For example, by having an item dedicated in memory of the child, the child can continue some form of eternal presence in the world. Others may contribute to a church nursery in memory of the child. All of these examples move the loss from a state of emptiness, destruction, and incompletion to a state of material being, helpfulness, and completion. The new state moves the loss to a place where the loss can be approached. The griever can then approach and react to the loss.

A Need to Find a Reason for the Loss

A "reason" is different from a "meaning." A reason gives the event cause. A meaning gives the event reaction. A reason does not move the loss but instead makes it approachable. While this can have dangerous side effects, some grievers will insist on creating a cause. Even though some perceived causes may have no connection to reality, the holder will still protect the cause as it serves a necessary end.

Sometimes, partners will have different reasons for the pregnancy loss. The different reasons may have temporal or eternal characteristics. For example, a bereaved mother may discover a satisfying reason for a pregnancy loss in the air pollution where she lives. Her partner may find his reason for the same loss in God's punishment for having had sex before marriage. Both partners will usually be able to coexist in harmonious relationship even with contrasting reasons as long as the "reason" is not imposed upon others.

One who discovers a reason for pregnancy loss may discover some hidden dangers in the result. Pastoral caregivers need to help grievers find constructive paths through their reasons. It is not the goal of pastoral care to take away the reason, even if it is potentially destructive. An example of a "destructive reason" would be that someone did something wrong to "deserve" the loss. A destructive reason such as this is not unusual in light of grievers' likelihood to be highly introspective and to be low on rationality. This type of reason often forces grievers to "put blood on someone's hands" and give them blame for the loss. This direction is extremely dangerous for the healing process in grief. For example, one person who suffered pregnancy loss remembered a grandmother warning her that God would not bless her marriage since she married outside of the family faith. This woman blamed herself and held her husband's existence as cause for the death. This did not lead toward grief healing. However caregivers may try, they seldom will "talk the person out of their reason." It would be more successful to help the person work his or her way through the reason and, hopefully, allow the person to see its flaws.

Another danger can occur when individuals wish to impose a reason upon a griever. For example, a well-intentioned person may give a cause such as, "it would have been handicapped and been a problem to you, so God saved you the hurt." The individual may find this offensive to his or her parenting skills. Imposition of these reasons can be destructive to the person who is not receptive to this particular reason. Generally, the griever is an easy victim for such an imposition as he or she is often in a low energy state and not able to maintain proper boundaries. Some in the church may wish to impose an "answer" to "defend" a God who seemed very incompetent in protecting the baby. It is helpful not to allow such people to impose these needs upon the griever. Romans 8:28, "All things work together for good to those who love God" is an often used verse for persons wishing to impose their values. Well-intentioned people will minister to the griever by attempting to impose a "good" that may have come from the loss and, as in an earlier case study in Chapter 2, justify God for allowing the baby to die. This is meaningful to the well-intentioned person, but it does not help the griever. The "good reasons" seldom make sense to the griever.

A third danger can occur when reasons for the loss, whether imposed or not, come into conflict with other reasons or values. A well-intentioned person may tell the griever that, "God took your child because He wanted an angel in heaven." This reason may be very meaningful to one individual and yet be terribly offensive to another. Some may become angry at God for being so insensitive as to kill a child for His personal needs. That reason can be very much in conflict with values held by another.

The spiritual journey that results from these needs can be long and painstaking. This requires that caregivers need to be patient with those on this journey. Caregivers need to let the person make their journey without interference. Often, caregivers who interfere to help shorten the journey only make the journey longer when the person has to come back and retrace necessary steps that the caregiver removed.

For example, the caregiver may be very aware that there are no "reasons" for most pregnancy losses. Very few pregnancy losses ever have a medical explanation. In spite of that, some will seek "reasons" even though there is no possibility of such discovery. The person will travel countless dead-end roads trying to discover the hidden reason. Unfortunately, any attempt to cut off a griever's search for reason will only make the person more determined and more secretive in his or her search. The process will only take longer and the caregiver will be removed as a resource for support. More effective ministry is found when the caregivers make themselves available to support the griever in these journeys—even if such ventures appear pointless to the caregiver.

Further problems along the journey can occur if the environment is not supportive for the spiritual endeavor. For example, one seeking a "reason" for loss may undertake a study of medical books in search of answers that were "unable to be discovered by physicians." Others may find themselves in extended prayer time seeking "God's reason" for the loss. These people may be distracted from their employment or other responsibilities. The ones to whom these responsibilities are owed may not be receptive to the failure to meet obligations. The caregiver may be useful in helping grievers develop negotiating skills with their environment to allow maximum time upon their spiritual journey.

In addition to these possible needs, there may be questions upon which the griever will focus. Few of these questions ever will have an "answer." Usually the seeker will know that before the question is ever raised. However, the griever may pursue these questions and other questions as a necessary endeavor in the grief process. Common questions are:

1. Why did God choose my baby?
2. Why did God never act while my baby was dying?
3. Why couldn't the physicians do more to save my child?
4. What could I have done to save my child?
5. Why must I say, "Good-bye?"
6. How can I learn to let go of my child?

These questions may take an enormous amount of time in the pursuit of answers. While this pursuit may appear fruitless, it has great meaning for the griever. From experience, only grievers will know when they have completed their journey.

PRACTICAL MINISTRIES AT PREGNANCY LOSS

There are many forms of ministry that can be provided by any members of virtually any local church. Some of these are practical ministries that do not require significant training for implementation. The major prerequisite for such ministries is a compassionate spirit. Expertise in ministry can be performed not only by outside sources such as trained medical or counseling staff.

The following lists include some forms of ministry that a church can provide. These are not intended to be exhaustive lists. They may serve best as suggested options that open the opportunity for each church's own ministry repertoire.

Developing a Protective Wall

While the caregiver needs to allow grievers freedom in seeking their way through the grief journey, total freedom is not the ultimate goal. Since the population experiencing pregnancy is generally a younger group than the average population, the sufferers of pregnancy loss will enter the grief with less than "a lifetime of wisdom." In addition, the grief experience will make the griever extremely vulnerable. The setting is very dangerous for the griever. It would be irresponsible pastoral care to never give opinions if the caregiver spotted the griever entering into harmful settings. In some situations, caregivers need to do more than give opinions; they need to create protective walls.

By a "protective wall," it is meant that the persons experiencing a loss are protected against making the loss multiply into further disaster. While this should be obvious, many caregivers overlook this ministry. Often it is neglected because the caregiver assumes that the person will not do anything of further harm. It is assumed that grievers, while experiencing pain from grief, will be especially aware of further hurt and protect themselves. In reality, this assumption is false.

Like the panicking animal in a forest fire that runs directly into the flames, so people who experience grief will often make poor decisions that only magnify the damage. It is important that caregivers are aware of this possibility and help prevent further damage through use of a "protective wall." Most grievers, wounded from their hurt, will welcome such support if the counselor knows when to withdraw the wall at an appropriate rate that returns personal rights to the griever. It is important that the only purpose for the wall be to keep harm from coming in and not to keep the person from experiencing freedom.

A biblical model for this ministry is found in Job 1:10, where Satan is unable to hurt Job because a protective hedge has been placed around Job. While there is no explanation of the quality of the hedge, it becomes apparent that the hedge is able to keep Job from harm. While the caregiver's wall, or hedge, will not match one provided by Divine Order, it will be helpful nonetheless.

Walls include both immediate protection and long-term protection. Immediate protection prevents grievers from inflicting any immediate damage to themselves or others. For example, if the pregnancy loss occurs at a hospital, the caregiver is responsible to be sure that grievers do not attempt to drive home while in a state of disorientation. Medical personal should be employed if there may be any doubt of the driving capacities of the grievers. Failure of caregivers to build such a protective wall can only risk an already destructive situation turning into a multiple tragedy.

Some grievers may begin to verbalize in a manner that will not lead to a healing of grief. Some grievers will begin to accuse others around them or will begin confessing all sorts of behaviors. This may be helpful to the griever at the moment but will only create further long-term problems. A number of protective walls, such as letting the person speak to a trained counselor in private, can be extremely helpful.

Long-term walls include encouraging grievers to avoid making any major life decisions while in grief. There is an odd desire on the part of many grievers to make major irreversible changes in their lives at the height of their grief. Some examples may be: to leave their employment, to change careers, to quit school, to leave their marriage, or to move to another location. These sudden changes often lead to additional problems, including but not limited to serious financial crisis, which will keep the person from facing his or her grieving needs and only postpone the healing.

A further issue needs to be addressed. Some people, while under stress, will make unrealistic promises to God that only cause future difficulties in their lives. A model of this can be found in Judges 12:30-39 where Jephthah ends up having to deny his daughter the privilege of marriage because of a rashly made vow. Caregivers need to use sensitivity in providing counsel. The caregiver needs to maintain the highest ethics as there may be a conflict of interest in such vows. For example, the griever may make an unrealistic financial vow to God that would benefit the caregiver's church. The caregiver must be sure that there are no compromises of Christian values in exchange for a potential personal gain. Either way, these vows are made under tremendous duress and should be treated as any other statements made in such a moment of crisis.

There are risks in placing protective hedges. Most other professions will avoid this ministry because it can appear to be a "control" over another that can later lead to a lawsuit and embarrassing charges. The church should feel comfort in providing this ministry if common sense is employed. The simplest rule is to suggest rather than to control. The counselor should make suggestions before witnesses who can verify the nature of the ministry. If the persons appear to be a danger to themselves or others, avoid making any ministries that could be considered "controlling" without first gaining support from other professionals. If members of other professions will not support you in such ministry, give strong consideration to abandoning the plan.

Providing Touch and Personal Experience

Many grievers can benefit from the privilege of seeing and even making physical contact with the deceased. This is especially true in pregnancy loss. Much of this ministry will be initiated by medical staff. The pastoral caregiver can be of effective use as a support person for this ministry. However, in some settings, medical personnel will be unavailable for such initiation. Pastoral caregivers can take the lead in providing this ministry.

It has long been known that parents who are able to see and touch their deceased babies are able to make effective use of grief time.

> Glen Davidson (1977) conducted a 5-year study of mothers who suffered a stillbirth or neonatal death. He discusses ways the women and the people around them coped with the loss of the child. Davidson describes the process by which the mothers in his study tried to move from disorientation to orientation. There were three points at which they were thwarted: first, when trying to confirm their loss perceptually; second, when reaching out for emotional support; and third, when trying to test their feelings against the perceptions of others. Davidson found that perceptual confirmation of having given birth is a crucial part of women's becoming reoriented after the baby's death. Those women who held and touched their babies, even at the moment of death, were found to adapt to their loss more successfully than those who had not.[1]

> In a study of 29 couples who had experienced stillbirth: Only six couples did not see their babies. Four of the mothers in these cases had undergone D&Cs, so the fetuses were dismembered. However, the fifth mother who underwent a D&C asked that her baby be pieced back together again so that she could see it![2]

The personal touch brings grief into an arena where grievers can experience the reality of loss. In this arena grievers can put limitations upon their loss and find the means to develop strategies for grief resolution.

There are many barriers that hinder medical or mortuary staff from offering this opportunity to touch the deceased baby. The same reluctance may also be found on the part of the pastoral caregiver. The caregiver will often personally feel very uncomfortable in experiencing the reality of the death and assume that he or she is providing a service by protecting the family from having to touch the baby. The caregiver may also fear that parents will "lose it" if they see their baby. The caregiver may think that the baby will look repulsive and, therefore, assume that viewing the baby will be detrimental to successful grieving.

From experience, these problems seldom happen. Parents seldom notice imperfections in their children. Instead, parents who are allowed to see their deceased babies will focus away from any physical defects and see the parts of the baby that are most attractive. The expected fears of the staff seldom, if ever, occur. The much more likely possibility is that the staff person will later hear the family report the experience to be the most meaningful way to begin healing their grief.

While many contemporary caregivers are afraid of parents seeing and touching their deceased baby, experience shows that the greater danger comes from parents who are denied this privilege. Without such an opportunity, the family may be left to imagine how their baby may have looked. Imagination can be more detrimental to successful grieving than actually viewing the baby since imagination can create a more frightening experience than would be found in reality. Parents of miscarriage and stillbirth, especially, may find themselves imagining a horrible creature that was more repulsive than could be found in any real birth defects. They will be pleased to know how wrong they are. Some parents will appreciate having a blanket to cover any parts of the babies body that may have imperfections. This may be helpful if there is significant discoloration due to difficulty in delivery or an extended time in the womb in stillbirth. This option allows the parents to open the blanket to their level of comfort. The blanket will be made more appropriate for presentation if placed in a microwave or other form of warmer before wrapping the baby.

The manner of the presenter is extremely important. The person presenting the baby needs to first ask the family if they wish to view the baby. If the family desires to do so, the presenter needs to develop a level of comfort in the act of presentation. The simplest manner of presentation is to present the baby as one would any other baby. For example, the baby should be held close to the presenter's body and maintained in a protective manner typical of any other baby.

Usually the mother will be the one most receptive for the baby. If she seems uncomfortable or lacks receptiveness, the baby can be presented to the father whose acceptance can prepare the mother to receive her baby. Sometimes neither the mother nor the father will feel comfort in receiving the baby, particularly if it is the couple's first child. To make the family more receptive, the presenter needs to patiently display the baby like any other newborn and model the level of comfort that they hope the family will develop. The presenter can point out the parts of the baby that deserve note in a normal newborn. For example, in a live birth the parents normally check the baby out by counting fingers and toes. If the baby is developed enough to do so, the presenter can show the family that all the fingers and toes are intact. If the baby is not so developed, the presenter can show the parent other features such as the nose, legs, ears, etc. The presenter can then gently encourage the family to touch the baby. Eventually, the family will usually become comfortable with holding the baby.

Once the baby is presented to the family, the presenter should step away from the family. This act will communicate to the family that they are in control of the baby. However, the presenter should remain nearby in case the family should need support. If the family is comfortable with holding their baby, the presenter can then leave the family in the same manner as if presenting a live child. As with a living child, the presenter or other medical staff person should be available for help or other support.

There is no direct rule for the proper length of time for the family to hold the baby. While the "normal" length is from twenty minutes to an hour, some families may have different needs. The longest request known to the author was in a setting where the family asked to have their baby for over eight hours. The family used the setting as a funeral visitation. Many family and friends were called in by the parents for a chance to help them begin their grief. While this is most unusual, it neither created any significant problems for the hospital staff nor challenged any hospital policies. It did, however, make the work of the funeral director more difficult and would have required a closed casket had a formal funeral been desired.

These moments of support to a family while they touch their child may prove emotionally difficult for some caregivers. It is not unprofessional for these caregivers to shed tears. Unless the caregiver is likely to completely lose control, it is usually better to allow the hurt to be expressed than to appear insensitive by faking apathy. The author's only awareness of a caregiver expressing tears leading to a problem involved a nurse who experienced unresolved grief from her own pregnancy loss.

In helping hospital or other staff experience grief, the pastoral caregiver enters into the larger task of ministry. It should not be assumed that the family will be the only ones present with spiritual needs. Often medical staff members will have extreme difficulty with the loss. They may experience all sorts of feelings of fear and guilt and find themselves grieving the loss quite acutely. It is also wrongly assumed that skilled medical professionals such as physicians will not need pastoral care at such a setting. Some medical personnel will experience feelings of professional failure in addition to their feelings of grief. The pastoral caregiver needs to be aware of all whose needs may come from the loss.

Providing Options for the Family

Most families who experience pregnancy loss have little to no awareness of options that are available to them. They often become passive, assuming that the professional staff will know how to care for their loss. Unfortunately, that same professional staff often will hesitate to provide options until the family expresses a need. The result is that very few options are presented, and the family will leave an institutional setting with little ministry beyond the core level.

Whether the setting is a hospital, funeral home, or church, the pastoral care team can present a full collection of options to a family suffering from pregnancy loss. The caregiver can use a chart that lists choices with specific details that are available to the family. That chart should not be presented in an impersonal manner. Before presenting the chart, the caregiver should provide a personal presentation of the main details of each service. The personal presentation provides supportive answers that avoid unnecessary stress for a family that already has many other stresses.

Many caregivers are afraid of presenting options; they have two fears that need to be faced. The first fear is that presenting options will offend people who are not willing or who are unable to grieve. This seldom, if ever, actually occurs. People will be very appreciative of options because they provide the grieving family with an element of control in an otherwise out-of-control setting.

The second fear is that too many options will be confusing. Theoretically, this should be a concern. Grievers do not have much energy for details and would likely become overwhelmed by a large collection of options. However, in practice, most grievers are able to quickly sort through options that do not meet their needs and focus upon the ones in which they have interest. Neither of these fears ever poses a serious problem.

The unseen danger of presenting options comes in losing objectivity in the presentation. Many caregivers unknowingly find themselves imposing options. Caregivers will often bring their comfort level into the presentation and find themselves influencing the choices. Probably, other professionals will have already placed grief values upon these grieving families. For example, not all funeral directors will allow a funeral for an unborn baby. Not all hospitals allow parents to see their deceased child. Pastoral caregivers can easily find themselves joining such an approach. Instead, caregivers need to develop a level of comfort beyond their specific personal preferences. In so doing, the caregiver can present the grieving family with options that will appear reasonable and would be helpful in their grief recovery. No families will likely be offended with options being presented unless the presenter totally lacks sensitivity. If families are allowed to refuse ministries, they still will appreciate the options being presented.

Specific Options That Are Available

Any church can provide a number of specific options for those who suffer from pregnancy loss. These ministry options do not require extended training, finances, or other resources. The difficulty for most churches comes in giving themselves comfort and permission to end the long precedent of not providing such options. If this can be overcome, new ministries become available.

Specific Option: Baptism/Dedication. Depending upon the theology of the institution, a ministry of baptism or dedication can provide the grieving family with significant support. Some theologies will insist that only a dedication can be provided for a miscarried or stillborn child. In that case, the child can be dedicated in a manner as close to the baptism ritual as the caregiver chooses to use. There are a number of rituals available that are specific for a dedication of the baby who has died due to pregnancy loss. If the baby is born alive but death is imminent, the hospital staff will generally be allowed to perform a baptism. Staff members of a church may use that emergency baptism to integrate with their own religious baptism provided later should the child survive.

The controversial use of baptism/dedication can be minimized by placing the choice in the hands of the parents. If the parents request the baptism/dedication, a staff member can perform the service. A simple ritual can include:

Opening Statements:	Explain the meaning of the service. Invite any available hospital staff and family to join.
Readings:	Psalm 139:13-16; Mark 10:13-16 can be helpful.
Prayer:	Heavenly God, creator and giver of all life, we come before you with questions, hurts, and even doubts. But most important, we come into your presence with a common love for this child of yours. We have yet to say, "Hello" and

now must say, "Good-bye." We are not prepared to say either.

In these moments, remind us that we, like this child, are loved by you and are promised your place when this world can no longer house our spirit.

As you received children into your bosom when you were on the earth, receive this child into your tender care, and receive our request that we may find the means of releasing him/her into a better place. May we so live our lives that we, too, may one day be joined together in that place where death can no longer separate us. We pray in Christ's name. Amen.

Consecration: (Name) I dedicate/baptize you into God's everlasting care. May the privileges of God's Grace abide in your life. Amen.

Benediction: As God's love has come into all of us, may we so find Grace in our life to continue the wonderful celebration of life that has been placed in our midst, now and forever more. Amen.

Providing Memorial Items

An outstanding form of ministry occurs in allowing the family members to collect memorial items by which they can remember their lost child. Almost all families will greatly appreciate any type of remembrance of their lost babies. This should be a standard procedure in the church. Babies who die should be remembered at Memorial Day or other times as any other person who has died. The only exception, a major concern of confidentiality, is found among those who do not want the news of their pregnancy to become public knowledge. The simplest way to avoid this problem is to set a policy that no memorial messages will be released until the knowledge of the pregnancy has been made public or that special permission is granted for the church to make it public.

Another way to help families find healing in their grief is to let them take home items used at the hospital or funeral service. In all cases, memorial items should be kept confidential and released only to the family. If the family should choose to not receive the memorials, experience encourages that the items should be kept by the church or other institution in a confidential place. Many family members will desire the mementos six months to a year after their loss. Keeping the memorials requires only minimal space and difficulty. However, if there is a risk of confidentiality violation, a church is best advised to dispose of the unclaimed memorial items immediately.

Usually, the hospital will initiate the items for a baby book. However, not all hospitals will do so, particularly in pregnancy loss. In that case, a church can begin the process. The church need only keep on file any church mementos that would involve the birth of the baby. For example, newsletters or Sunday bulletins may have a mention of planned baby showers, birth announcements, and sympathy notes. These are helpful items to include in a memorial packet.

If the hospital is providing a memorial book, the pastoral caregiver can add to the process. By involving either the hospital or the funeral director, if the latter is used, memorial items can be collected involving the baby's body. A picture, footprints, a lock of hair, any items from the baby isolette, items from the dedication/baptism, and items used for baby identification can be collected and included in a memorial packet. Any other items that would normally be put in a packet for a living baby can be used in the setting of pregnancy loss. Generally, the family need only to request that these options be provided to initiate the process. However, the pastoral caregiver often will need to empower the family to request the materials. Note: make sure the griever does not interpret "empower" to mean "coerce." The pastoral caregiver can also provide institutional personnel with details of specific items to be placed in the memorial packet.

Persons uninvolved in stillbirth experiences might be repulsed by the idea of collecting memorabilia, (as well as seeing and holding the baby), but it is the standard practice in competent handling of such situations today. The invaluable keepsakes help in capturing the depth of love and loss, and in enhancing the grieving process itself.[3]

The only major obstacle for such ministry can occur when funeral or medical personnel become uncooperative. Some such professionals still feel that pregnancy loss is best grieved when the loss is ignored. Even with progress being made in many other areas of the two professions, there are still some who feel this way. The family needs to insist on their rights as the parents of the child if the hospital or funeral director do not cooperate.

Naming the Baby

Giving a child a name would appear to be a simple act that should be provided to all babies. However, this is not to be assumed the case. In many cases of pregnancy loss, many do not name their baby simply because the option is never presented. While some may choose not to name their baby, many are pleased with the opportunity to do so. Many find significant help in their grieving by giving their child a name. The process of giving a name to the baby allows the family to identify their loss. It will also give dignity to the baby by giving it the same dignity as any other baby would receive.

The decision to name a baby need not be made immediately. In any birth, the child is not always named right after delivery. Especially with the stress of the medical problems, some families simply cannot decide upon a name. If there is any difficulty, the family can give the child a name at any later point in time. If there is a death certificate, the changes, if desired, can be made at a later date as well.

If the baby dies from an early miscarriage and the sex of the child is not determined, several options for naming remain available. Some families choose to name the child a unisex name such as, "Pat," "Terry," or "Bobby." Others may use intuitive feelings and assign the sex to the baby and give the baby a gender-appropriate name.

We strongly encourage you to give your baby a name, preferably the name you had been planning for the child all along. Don't "save" the name for your next child. It rightly belongs to this one.

Names are important. You will use the name as you talk about this little person to others. You will use it as you tell your other children about this special child in your life. You will find it easier to connect your memories to this child if you can refer to him or her by name.[4]

Funeral Ministries

The idea of people grieving their lost babies is not new. It is also not new to provide some form of burial ministry. In American cemeteries, it is not unusual to see baby graves that are over a century old. Even creative ways to memorialize a pregnancy loss are not new. For example, the "Baby Ruth" candy bar commemorates the death of former President Grover Cleveland's baby, Ruth, who died in newborn loss many years ago. Grief has brought some very creative means of memorializing in other ways as well.

For some reason, we appear to have recently lost that ability. Perhaps it is because the majority of babies are no longer born at home where the family had to see and experience the loss. In our recent era, bodies of babies, whether born or miscarried, are often disposed by being dumped in garbage disposal-like instruments. Some hospitals still dump the smaller babies into a toilet. The technician who performs the disposal will seldom have any personal contact with the family of loss. This new convenient process insulates us from the experiences that nurture this creativity. In many ways this hinders our ability to grieve.

Many find this convenience far from appropriate. We would not consider this type of disposal as an option for bodies of older family members when they die. Many parents find the current "normal" method to be terribly inadequate for their child.

The faith community can provide an alternative. The alternative is in the dignity of a funeral. This option allows the family to use the normal means of grief to work through their loss. There may also be a burial for babies who die from pregnancy loss. This provides the family with a place to face their grief in a very tangible manner. These become excellent tools toward successful grief work.

However, a word of caution is in order. Beginning a ministry of funerals for pregnancy loss is not always properly appreciated. The clergy who initiates the ministry is open to all sorts of strange accusations. These accusations can prove to be awkward for many clergy who feel that their integrity needs to be kept above reproach. Generally, the worst charge will be that the pastor is exploiting other's grief for financial gain. These charges will come from well-meaning people who find pregnancy loss best grieved through denial and avoidance. They are troubled that a pastor would circumvent that process. Even though funerals for pregnancy loss generate little to no income for a pastor or a funeral director and often are provided at a financial loss, the charge will be hard to fight. However, both clergy and funeral director will consider the "negative connotation" well compensated by the extreme positive responses of those families who request a funeral.

Finding a ritual for a pregnancy loss is no longer difficult. In 1985 there were very few from which to choose. By the early 1990s many denominations had developed a ritual for the funeral of a pregnancy loss. Many funeral directors also have numbers of ecumenical rituals for clergy who are unable to find one that meets their need.

When serving in a chaplain setting, things can be more complex. The family of loss may be of another faith. Depending upon the level of comfort, there are many things that can be done even when the family does not share a common faith. For example, many faiths will recognize a chaplain's blessing upon a death. The Aaronic Blessing of Numbers 6:24-26 can often be used in a multicultural setting:

The Lord bless you and keep you;
the Lord make his face shine upon you and be gracious to you;
the Lord lift up his countenance upon you and give you peace.

(King James Version)

If, as chaplain, you are requested to contact a representative of the individual's faith for a funeral or other care, it is helpful to be as supportive as possible. Each faith will be different. For example, if the person is an Orthodox Jew, the rabbi will have difficulty in providing a funeral for the pregnancy loss. However, a rabbi of the Reformed Jewish faith may be able to provide the care. It is important to work with the faith leader even if he or she seems uncooperative. Often they are under obligations of which they cannot compromise but will help direct you to people who can provide the service. In many situations, you may be tempted to step in yourself and provide the care. While it may solve the immediate problem, this is a dangerous step. Unlike the local church, as chaplain, it is unprofessional to circumvent the individual's faith setting. In any case, do not "burn the bridges" behind the family of loss by damaging their relationship with the body that will be needed for their faith support at such a vulnerable time.

Many suggest that a childlike atmosphere can add to the quality effect of the funeral. Any items that keep the baby casket from becoming a "sterile object" will serve well. For example, placing baby toys around the casket can present the baby in such a manner that people will sense comfort as they come close to the baby. Some funeral directors are able to make the entire funeral home appear like a children's day care center or nursery for funerals involving pregnancy loss. Some clergy consider this atmosphere to compromise the religious message and impact of the funeral. If so, the childlike setting can be used at a visitation. In addition to inviting grievers into an experience with the loss, this atmosphere is generally considered to be less intimidating to children who might wish to attend the funeral.

When planning a funeral for a baby, some parents have included:

- Baby music played over the funeral home sound system.
- Balloons in the room.
- Stuffed toys.
- A letter to your baby from the two of you, written together, or a letter from each of you which can be read by yourself, the clergyperson, or a friend of your choice.

- A simple, traditional service might feel right for you, or a personal, less formal gathering might be all you want.
- If you have other children, you may want to let them see the baby, touch if they want, or put a memento into the casket.[5]

A final option can be made available to the parent. During the visitation, the parent(s) could hold the baby while people come by to visit. Even if the baby was held for a few moments by a parent, the act could be helpful in bringing reality to the grief. Even with the progress that we have made thus far, this is a bold step. Such an act that brings the reality of loss to onlookers may not be appreciated by some. A suggested means of preparing people for this act would be to announce to the group who may be conversing at the visitation that "In five minutes the mom will bring the baby out of the casket for them to touch, if they would like to do so." An announcement such as that will prepare those who wish to distance themselves from the event to find a comfortable location.

Most people are surprised to discover the number of options that are available for a burial involving a pregnancy loss. While each state has different regulations, all have relaxed requirements regarding burial when pregnancy loss is involved. Some states do not require a vault or that the body be buried more than two feet below the surface. This option can be helpful for friends or family who wish to provide support but feel unable to do so. If the cemetery does not have restrictions, in pregnancy loss, anyone can help dig the grave. There are not the limitations as in other losses requiring special equipment and vaults. Those who have provided these labors of love report that it relieves their feelings of helplessness in wanting to lend aid, yet feel unable to discover a means to carry out that aid.

While pregnancy loss provides many more burial options due to lack of restrictions, it also provides less expensive options. For example, many cemeteries have children's sections in which gravesite costs are available at a fraction of the costs for other sites. This is crucial in that pregnancy loss usually comes at a time when the parents do not have the financial resources to purchase a full-expense site. Also, pregnancy loss often occurs at a time when the parents are not sure of long-term location and often have given no consideration to where their own burial site would best be located.

Choosing a less expensive children's gravesite allows the parents time to select a large lot for themselves and have the child later moved into that lot with a fraction of the expense of an adult transfer. As in any such moves, state and cemetery regulations need to be followed. It is recommended that this be done by a funeral director who has experience in this area. Such individuals can save the family endless amounts of work and expense.

NOTES

1. Rando, T.A. *Parental Loss of a Child.* Champaign, IL: Research Press Company, 1986, p. 76.

2. Fickling, K.F. "Stillborn Ministries: Ministering to Bereaved Parents." *The Journal of Pastoral* Care, (47) 3. (Fall 1993): 222.

3. Ibid., p. 220.

4. Schwiebert, P., RN and P. Kirk, MD. *When Hello Means Goodbye.* Burnsville, NC: Rainbow Connection, 1993, p. 19.

5. Lister, M., and S. Lovell. *Healing Together—For Couples Grieving the Death of Their Baby.* Burnsville, NC: Rainbow Connection, p. 2.

Chapter 8

Ministries After a Pregnancy Loss

"Aftercare" is a term used for the support of bereaved persons following the funeral service. Traditionally, many disciplines ceased to provide care once the funeral had been completed, assuming that the needs of the bereaved family were fulfilled after the funeral committal. In recent years, a major change has occurred in most of the caring disciplines. It is becoming clear to most of these disciplines that the task of most bereavement services is just beginning with the funeral. These disciplines have noted that the living are not able to begin caring for themselves until the funeral is over. Grievers are not able to discover the problems of "life alone" until after the funeral is finalized. At this time the grievers will begin to identify and experience their points of grief. Grief points can be divided into two parts: (1) crisis issues and (2) long-term adjustments. It is often wise to also divide the grief support task into these two departments. While such a division will break up the continuity of care by using more than one person, for practical reasons it is essential for the support system to separate the two tasks. Crisis problems, which can occur at any given time of day, require immediate care. The person providing long-term care cannot continually be available to the twenty-four-hour ministry of crisis support. Such caregivers will "burn out" rather quickly. Crisis support people need to serve for short periods of time with significant opportunities for "time away." By the time long-term support is necessary, the griever will be less likely to need twenty-four-hour support. The long-term support caregiver can afford to maintain his or her regular hours by providing scheduled support meetings. Needs for long-term support in pregnancy loss may include needs such as financial issues, medical issues, support in planning for a subsequent pregnancy, facing holidays, and facing the general public, among other issues. The crisis caregiver can often be trained by local professionals at very little cost to the church. Long-term support caregivers often become more effective as a care coordinator, with emphasis upon knowing whom to refer rather than trying to take on all the tasks themselves. In either crisis or long-term support, it is extremely crucial that caregivers know limitations of their skills and know the resources to employ when the grief needs are beyond their care abilities.

CRISIS MINISTRY SUPPORT

For many persons who experience pregnancy loss, there are many crisis issues that occur from time to time. Often, there are no solutions to the crisis problems. The grieving person simply needs someone to hear his or her hurt expressions. The crisis counselor can be most effective in simply helping grieving persons solve their own crisis by using their own best judgment. For example, those who think they are "going crazy" can receive ministry by allowing themselves to evaluate their own grief compared to the setting and determine if the grief reaction is a significant psychiatric problem or is simply a normal grief response. If a griever feels that his or her grief is not normal, it would be wise to provide reference to a professional caregiver. Often grievers will simply be frightened by their grief experience and merely need someone to hear their hurt. In most cases, grievers will indicate that the grief is not unusual, and the trained support person will see no danger in the immediate future. Unfortunately, this process will often require significant amounts of resource time. Crisis support people need to be individuals who can provide significant patience in their ministry. This filtering process can be very helpful as long as the caregiver errs on the side of getting help rather than ignoring serious problems.

Adding to the stress of crisis counseling, much of the grief work is slow and repetitive. The griever often finds themselves taking "one step backward for every two steps forward." While this leads to long-term progress, usually the crisis support person only sees the "backward step." This setting can create stress for the support person. For this reason, crisis support workers need to avoid providing long-term care. Instead, they should allow themselves some self-care time in between crisis care cases.

LONG-TERM SUPPORT

Long-term support can be entirely different from crisis care. The experienced support person will be very helpful to the griever by anticipating problems and by beginning to solve problems before they occur. This anticipation takes much of the emotional crisis from the problem both for the griever and the caregiver. Anticipation also allows grievers to prepare themselves with options to face the potential crisis. Here are some of the grief points to anticipate:

Support in Facing Holidays

The term "holidays" refers to any special gathering, usually involving family-oriented events, in which grief can be acute. Often, Thanksgiving, Christmas, and New Year's Day are days that can cause significant crisis in the griever. Any one such crisis will lead to significant backward steps in the grief process.

These holidays will often create strong emotions of family-oriented blessings and celebration. To an individual who has recently suffered pregnancy loss, symbols of blessing such as a Thanksgiving Prayer, presents under a Christmas tree, or best wishes for a new year, can be strong reminders of the missing person and the huge void left by the loss. Persons can enter the holidays feeling very much in emotional control only to be suddenly overcome by grief. These sudden attacks can be unbearable.

The long-term support system can help the griever by warning of the potential problem and providing techniques that can minimize the impact from "holiday grief." The warning is extremely helpful in that grievers will often find themselves feeling forms of acute grief that, at first, will seem inappropriate for the setting. This can lead to denial, which leads to more vulnerability or concerns of personal sanity when the grief develops. When the long-term support worker provides grievers with awareness of the grief potential, grievers will be able to emotionally "brace themselves" for a grief experience that, hopefully, will not happen.

Simple techniques can minimize the impact of holiday grief. Families going through their first year after pregnancy loss should schedule their holiday activities so that there is plenty of time for a grieving experience that may suddenly occur. For example, a couple who has recently experienced pregnancy loss can benefit greatly by not planning to host a major holiday gathering at their home. This does two things. First, the task of hosting a holiday gathering is often loaded with stress and creates a "busy" setting going into the holidays. Being busy often caps feelings of grief. Unfortunately, capping feelings often is like capping a volcano. The "capping" does not avoid the problem but, instead, only delays it until a much larger eruption occurs. Often, the large eruption will occur at a very inappropriate time, such as when the celebration is beginning and the hosting responsibilities are at a focal point. If the griever is not as busy, the grief attacks can come in lesser doses that are much easier to handle. Second, by not hosting the gathering grievers allow themselves to leave early, or not attend at all if they need time alone.

Another technique for dealing effectively with holiday grief is to schedule a time for the grief experience. For example, a visit to the grave with a holiday wreath can allow for helpful grief management. Some families have found it beneficial at Christmas to give a gift to an underprivileged child in the name of their lost child. These efforts can be very productive in allowing holiday grief to come in smaller, more manageable doses.

Support in Facing Due-Date Anticipation

Often, the expected date of baby delivery is many months later than the loss experience. In these situations, the family begins to get back to a reasonably normal life only to sense a sudden reversal when the due date arrives. When this happens, significant crisis can occur at the due date and temporarily reverse the grief healing process. The grieving family may think that they had progressed into their grief only to have a significant setback as the due date approaches.

The due date can bring a reality to the pregnancy loss. Many couples make this experience even more difficult by responding with "elephant in the room" behavior. The grief will be as big as an elephant but will not seem like it should exist. Since both parties are embarrassed to admit that they are experiencing this "elephant presence" they will pretend that it does not exist. Couples will go to tremendous effort to carry out the charade. If the couple will admit to and name their "elephant" they will feel tremendous relief. However, the size of the "elephant" grows bigger with every denial. If the couple is prepared for this experience, they can destroy the elephant by giving it an identity. At that point the elephant becomes very small and significantly less intimidating.

While there are many possibilities in making the due date more tolerable, such as taking time for self, no strategy can effectively remove the hurt. The best suggestions focus on "protecting the date" by not scheduling any important events, especially ones that would require a major attention focus. The good news is that due dates last only twenty-four hours. The grievers' lives can move on once this trying experience is over.

Support in Facing Future Anniversaries of Loss

Many of the same characteristics of the due date occur on annual anniversaries of loss. The first annual anniversary is often the worst anniversary. Many grievers indicate that there is a slow progression over the years when anniversaries come, with each having consistently less of an impact. It appears that caregivers do best to counsel with couples that they do not take any small regressions too seriously. The regressions from the normal progressions often occur with good reason. For example, the fifth year has a painful edge in that the child would be entering school. This creates a new level of grief. Family members realize that they no longer only grieve a baby but now must grieve the loss of a school-age child. Other potential dips or regressions often occur in grieving the beginning of the second decade of life, the grief of missing the child learning to drive, graduating from school, and getting married. Eventually there will be additional experiences of grief in missing the child presenting grandchildren and great-grandchildren.

The church can provide ministry by helping foster "elephant in the room" awareness. Many people appreciate receiving a "thinking of you" note at these difficult anniversaries. A personal contact such as a note or phone call allows the grievers a chance to feel support and an opportunity to share their grief. Getting the note provides an opportunity for the couples to identify the "elephant" that may return year after year.

There will be people who do not appreciate these contacts. They are people who are not able to work through their grief and prefer to avoid anything that will remind them of their loss. Such people will make themselves very clear of their displeasure in ministry attempts. Their requests should be respected.

Support During "Firsts"

Another similar area of difficulty that occurs with any loss is the experience of doing something for the first time after the loss. These "firsts" can be very traumatic. In addition to anniversary dates such as the beginning of school and graduations from school, all parents have to work through other new experiences of grief. They occur with the "first time" a person must take on an activity without his or her anticipated child. Some of these experiences, long after the funeral and when most ministry has concluded, can be very difficult experiences. There are numbers of "firsts" for each grieving couple. Some examples are: the first time returning to work, the first time back to church, the first time back to the clinic where prenatal care was received, the first time to hold another baby, and the first time to meet with friends and family, to name just a few examples. Also, the couple will have to face the guilt or other issues when they begin to have fun for the first time, be sexually intimate, and begin returning to a form of normal life. In addition to creating guilt, these experiences can be very lonely and depressing. Having a support person can be very helpful for the griever.

Support While Facing a World Insensitive to Pregnancy Loss

Unfortunately, much of the world is poorly equipped to respond to a family grieving from pregnancy loss. Insensitivity seems to be the rule rather than the exception when grievers begin returning to their world. Ministry is helpful in forewarning the grievers as to what they are going to face and in providing a place where the grievers can share their frustrations and hurts. Here are some areas that grievers in pregnancy loss can expect insensitivity.

Many new parents relate accounts of having all sorts of salespersons calling after their baby is born. Such sales organizations appear to watch local birth announcements and often respond rapidly with sales offers and promotional items. Unfortunately, these sales persons are trained to make sales and have little sensitivity for grieving families. Families should be forewarned about these types of callers and be prepared for incredibly insensitive contacts.

People who would be least expected to do so may make insensitive comments. Employers and even trained medical experts or church leaders have been recorded to make terribly inappropriate statements to grievers of pregnancy loss. It must be understood that there are many people who do not understand pregnancy loss. There are also some professionals that do not like babies. These people are capable of making the loss sound as if it were desired. The grievers are often hurt by these comments and are not able to understand that such comments only result from lack of understanding. While some find confrontation helpful in response to such people, often grievers can compound the problem by attempting to engage in the discussion. Ministry can be very helpful in supporting grievers through these difficult times.

Other people, with much better intentions, will cause all sorts of problems by "wanting to help." Unfortunately, many of their efforts are not helpful. Adding to the problem, the ones who are insisting on providing these unhelpful acts are often least likely to take the hint that their help is unwanted. While grievers do not have the energy to confront these individuals, wherever possible, ministry needs to avoid getting in the middle of such confrontations. Instead, ministry becomes more effective in empowering grievers to find ways to speak for themselves.

Another too often repeated setting occurs when insensitive people expect the griever to immediately, "get over" his or her grief. Because the insensitive person has had little experience with the pregnancy, that individual does not understand the reason behind the grief. Many such persons are beyond educating or changing. The griever needs to know that there will be plenty of such persons and that any comments from these persons need to be taken with little credence. The problem can be increased if these insensitive persons are in a power position such as an employer who cannot understand why the griever needs time away from work responsibilities. If the pregnancy loss is a newborn death, most state laws will allow for family leave. Unfortunately, few states will provide such support for stillbirths or miscarriages.

> The truth is that until you experience this terrible tragedy personally, you cannot know the right thing to say. People are trying to be helpful–they just don't know how to do it.[1]

Support in Facing Unanswerable Questions

Grievers often find themselves presented with questions that do not have answers. Instead of attempting to dismiss the questions or even trying to find answers, ministry can be more effective in working through the doubts. The support ministry can help by sorting out the various parts of these unanswerable questions. By breaking the questions into parts, resolution can be found by a "divide and conquer" method, assuming that a conquering point is accessible.

For example, parents who have undergone pregnancy loss may find themselves overwhelmed with their concerns whether or not they will ever see their baby in heaven. The mistake many caregivers make is to only provide the grieving person with church doctrine. While this may solve the immediate problem, it ignores the greater questions. Grievers often need to work through their doubts regarding an Almighty God who appeared to be passive while their child died. Grievers will need to work through their imagery of what their child would look like when they meet in heaven. Some parents want their child to be a baby forever. Others will want their child to grow into adulthood while in heaven. By helping persons work through their questions rather than reciting church doctrine, grievers can develop their own answers. Effective ministry teams often answer such questions with further, probing questions. "What do you think?" or "How do you imagine God working this out?" can be much more effective than simply discussing doctrine. Instead of using doctrine as an answer, use it instead to support the grievers' perceived answers. Doctrine does not help when used as a narrow track to hinder grief exploration.

Support in Preparing for Future Pregnancies

Eventually, most persons who suffer pregnancy loss will begin thinking of "trying again." Usually, they will feel the pain of loss subsiding but will not be sure they are ready to risk another loss. These persons will often want professionals to have an answer for them as to the proper time to begin the process. By the time they come to church for counsel, they usually have been to their obstetrician and various other medical experts. It is important that answers received from ministry be reasonably cohesive to the answers found in the medical community. This is one point where ministry workers may need to carefully avoid giving unhelpful "folk remedies." The couple will probably have heard plenty of such advice and are seeking some help in sifting through these remedies. If ministry workers do not have a researched reason for disagreeing with the medical community, they may do well to hold their opinions rather than further confuse the couple.

It would be helpful if there were a formula for parents to apply in knowing when they can feel comfortable about having another child after a pregnancy loss. Such a formula would say, "After (blank) time, you can safely think about having your next child." Unfortunately, no such formula exists. Couples generally do not need that formula. They seem to have a subjective sense of when they are prepared to begin another pregnancy. They need to empower themselves to be the final authority.

> Although there is little scientific evidence on this issue, it is often believed that those parents who have had more time to focus fully on the baby who has died, and who have had a fairly long gap before the conception of another baby, are likely to find another pregnancy and the development of their relationship with another baby less difficult.[2]

It is helpful to remind them that there will never be a time when they can be completely ready. It is also important to respect the feelings of the couple if they feel that they are not willing to try the risk again. Either way, it is extremely helpful if both the father and mother can have a mutual agreement in their progression.

When (or if) the time comes to try again, encourage the couple to select their obstetrician carefully. They will have many special needs. While all obstetricians are competent to care for their delivery, assuming it is not a high risk, not all will understand their personal needs. Sometimes special relationships develop between parents and medical staff that create superior trust. Professional obstetricians will not be offended if the couple finds that another competent physician is more helpful. It is wise for them to use their pastor among other friends and professionals to provide themselves with references to obstetricians who are likely to be most supportive to the personal needs. Encourage the couple to be specific in sharing their needs with a potential obstetrician.

> To get these things, I had to do some shopping around and be clear about my requirements. I tried to sift through some basic data by phone when I called for an appointment. Questions that the phone staff wouldn't answer and points I wanted to discuss with the doctor I wrote down and checked off during my initial office visit. This visit is much like an audition, and it is natural to feel a certain amount of embarrassment or self-consciousness but it is also important to overcome these feelings. We wouldn't dream of hiring other professionals, however specialized, without discussing the work involved. I think doctors need to be selected with equal care.[3]

OTHER SUPPORT MINISTRIES

Support for Numbering Family

While this may appear as a trivial issue to many, it is of significant importance to the family of loss. People are constantly asked, "Are you a parent?" or, "How many children do you have?" This is a part of the normal conversation within our society and is used toward formation of our identity. Individuals who have experienced pregnancy loss are never sure how to answer these questions, particularly if there are no surviving children. Each person must find an answer with which they will feel comfortable. Many simply need support in reaching that conclusion, especially if there is incongruence in the answer of the partner.

Special support is necessary for those who have experienced pregnancy loss and have no living children. These individuals will often feel as though they are parents but will forever be surrounded by strange responses when they respond in affirmation to the request, "Do you have children?" Some notorious answers that parents hear are, "But that doesn't count," or, "I mean *real* children." Sometimes it can be even worse when people completely stop talking following an affirmative answer. Many bereaved parents will begin to respond with a negative answer simply to avoid the bad experiences that may occur from a positive response.

Support for Grandparents' Needs

Grandparents often suffer a double hurt. They hurt from both their grief and their children's grief. They may add an additional hurt if the loss leads them to relive their own pregnancy loss experience from earlier years.

While grandparents may have significant needs, they are usually exempt from normal support systems. Because it may imply a breach of confidentiality, medical staff persons are often hesitant to answer questions raised by grandparents. Any grief support or ministry will focus on the immediate parents and ignore the needs of extended family. Grandparents often feel the need to care for their children, sometimes attempting to "rescue them from grief" by "being strong" rather than facing their own grief. This need can be reinforced by church or other support systems that overlook the needs of grandparents.

Instead of joining this setting of overlooking grandparents' needs or responding as if the needs were the same in the grief of parents, caregivers should understand the different focus of grandparents' grief. This can be discovered in various ways. Much like grieving parents, each grandparent brings unique needs that require unique ministry. In many situations, asking the grandparents how "they are doing" with an interest in the answer is effective in creating an open door for the bereaved to focus upon themselves and prepare for ministry. Sometimes grandparents find benefit through ministry that "names" the types of grief that grandparents can experience. This allows the grandparents to become aware of feelings that they are experiencing but are lacking ability to approach. Resolution can begin as the awareness makes the experience identifiable to them.

Pregnancy loss does readily have causes and "answers." Grandparents often understand this better than do their younger offspring. Ministry that presents "answers" or "reasons" for the loss is usually not appreciated by grandparents. Instead, an appreciation can be found in ministry that combines allowing the grandparents to discover their own "answers" or "reasons" and to find support where there are no answers and reasons.

Pregnancy loss equals loss of future. Grandparents feel this loss often more keenly than their children who may not yet understand their own finitude. Grandparents will place hope on grandchildren to "carry on" as they see their own end of life approaching. Grandparents may not be able to specifically name this grief and prefer that ministry not do so either. Naming the grief can be hurtful to grandparents for it forces recognition of their own death. Effective ministry should at most imply the need for future on earth after their own death rather than specifically name the immediate possibility of their death.

While many may attempt to provide sophisticated ministry, some of the most effective ministry for grandparents can occur by ministry presence. By ministry presence, this simply means "becoming available for ministry and providing a sense of concern and relationship toward the grandparent." Ministry presence brings the grandparents out of the cold and into contact with human beings who care that they are hurting. This is very similar to validating grief as occurred in a case study in Chapter 2. Ministry presence goes beyond validation and allows the grandparents to care for some of their needs. This presence allows the grandparents to express their hurts and frustrations toward their own resolution.

Support for Surviving Children

Surviving children present needs that are quite different from needs of parents and grandparents. Unlike grandparents, who can be denied information as a form of spite from unhappy children and in-laws, surviving children are often denied information by well-meaning people who think the lack of information can spare them hurt. Some have even advocated denying the surviving children the option of attending the funeral. This is seldom successful in helping children work through their grief. Sparing immediate hurt for these children only creates greater hurt at a later time. These children learn to suspect well-meaning people, which can include parents, medical staff, and pastors. Such learned suspicion creates greater, lifelong, problems.

> Studies have often shown that if a child's mourning cycle is repressed, the child may later react by internalizing these emotions in unhealthy ways, sometimes with the loss of the capacity for personal intimacy to show for it. "My parent abandoned me," reasons the child. "I'd better not get close to anyone else again or that person will do the same thing."[4]

There are numerous problems that frequently occur in surviving children who must respond to sibling death due to pregnancy loss. It is helpful for the caregiver to be aware of the needs that can arise from these problems. The children will seldom have opportunity to ever see or touch the lost sibling. This leads to an inability to identity with their grief. These children may also feel guilt from the loss.

Effective ministry to surviving siblings walks significant "tightropes." Ministry needs to avoid giving too much or too little information to the child. Too much information, even with parents' follow-through, adds to the confusion. Too little information frustrates the child. Children's questions should be answered wherever possible in as simple a manner as possible. Too much simplicity creates future problems. For example, to tell the surviving siblings that their brother or sister is "sleeping" will create a fear within the child toward sleep. To "blame" the loss on God will create a suspicion toward God.

Children do not expect adults to have answers to every question. Adults never have answers for their endless "Why" questions, such as, "Why is the sky blue?" and children learn to become comfortable with situations that have no answers. Children will understand that adults cannot answer all of their questions regarding the death of their siblings. Unfortunately, many adults tend to give children too simplistic an answer or brush off the question as being unimportant. These responses give the child very clear, but less than helpful answers.

Families who have experienced pregnancy loss may be difficult to minister to in some unexpected ways later on in life. Quite often staff workers in nursery or Sunday school will report significant difficulties with parents who seem to be very protective of their children. Not every time, but often, these parents will be ones who have lost a child in their past. These parents may not only resist any attempts to discipline their children, but will nearly deny the possibility that their children could do wrong.

Frustrated staff workers can compound the problem by ignoring or otherwise isolating these parents. Instead of this, they can be approached by much more effective means. Staff needs to understand the perspective that these parents bring into the setting. These parents treasure their children because they did not die, thus giving them hurt. They will protect their children in unusual ways as reward "for living." They will accept that their children can do wrong but will often first demand evidence. Instead of becoming frustrated with these parents, staff can initiate effective ministry by projecting a similar feeling of treasuring the children. Once that is communicated, the parents will become strong supporters of the staff.

SUMMARY

Grief from pregnancy loss requires sensitive and supportive care. Using the proper techniques and allowing the grieving person to provide direction for the care, including the power to reject ministry, can be helpful in creating this effective care. In their summary report involving 194 persons who have experienced pregnancy loss, Lasker and Toedter show that sensitivity and caring are crucial in meeting the needs of these grievers:

> In most cases, parents were more satisfied if they had experienced an intervention than if they had not, but having experienced more total interventions was not associated with lower grief or greater satisfaction with overall care; the latter was related more to the attentiveness and sensitivity of health care personnel.[5]

Unfortunately, many support groups assume that the griever from pregnancy loss either does not need ministry or that grief ministry should be provided as, "one size fits all." Quality ministry will come from those faith communities who are willing to match their gifts and skills with each unique need that comes to individuals suffering from pregnancy loss.

NOTES

1. Parrott, C., RN. *Parents' Grief: Help and Understanding After the Death of a Baby.* Redmond, WA: Medic Publishing Co., 1992, p. 18.

2. Kohner, N., and A. Henley. *When a Baby Dies.* San Francisco: Harper Collins Publishers, 1995, p. 123.

3. Pizer, H., and C. O'Brien Palinski. *Coping with a Miscarriage.* New York: Signet-New American Library, 1986, p. 158.

4. Carroll, D. *Living with Dying.* New York: Paragon House, 1991, p. 183.

5. Lasker, J.N., and L.J. Toedter. *Satisfaction with Hospital Care and Interventions After Pregnancy Loss.* Death Studies, 18:41-64, Washington, DC: Taylor and Francis, 1995, p. 41.

Appendix

Support Organizations

United States:

AMEND (Aiding a Mother Experiencing Neonatal Death)
4324 Berrywick Terrace
St. Louis, MO 63128
314-487-7582

Association for Recognition of Life of Stillbirths
11128 West Front Avenue
Littleton, CO 80127
303-978-9517

Centering Corporation
PO Box 3367
Omaha, NE 68103
402-553-1200

Compassionate Friends
PO Box 3696
Oak Brook, IL 60522
708-990-0010

DES Action USA
Long Island Jewish Hospital
New Hyde Park, NY 11040
1-800-337-9288

MIDS, Inc. (Miscarriage, Infant Death, Stillbirth)
16 Crescent Drive
Parsippany, NJ 07054
201-966-6437

National Maternal and Child Health Resource Center
2070 Chain Bridge Road
Suite #450
Vienna, VA 22182
703-821-8955

National Sudden Infant Death Syndrome Resource Center
2070 Chain Bridge Road
Suite #450
Vienna, VA 22182
703-821-8955

Perinatal Loss Project
2116 N.E. 18th Avenue
Portland, OR 97212-2621
503-284-7426

Pregnancy and Infant Loss Center
1421 East Wayzata Boulevard
Suite #30
Wayzata, MN 55391
612-473-9372

Pregnancy Loss Support Program
National Council of Jewish Women, NY Section
9 East 69th St.
New York, NY 10021
212-535-5900

RTS Bereavement Services
Lutheran Hospital-LaCrosse
1910 South Avenue
LaCrosse, WI 54601
1-800-362-9567 ext. 4747

SHARE ("A Source of Help in Airing and Resolving Experiences")
St. Joseph Health Center
300 First Capital Dr.
St. Charles, MO 63301
314-947-6164

SIDS Alliance
10500 Little Patuxent Parkway, Suite 420
Columbia, MD 21044
800-221-SIDS

Australia:

Compassionate Friends
Lower Parish Hall
300 Camberwell Road
Camberwell, Vic. 3124

SANDS (Stillbirth and Neonatal Death Support)
PO Box 708
South Brisbane, Qld.

United Kingdom:

Miscarriage Association
Clayton Hospital
Northgate, Wakefield
W. Yorks WF13JS

Scottish Cot Deaths Trust
Royal Hospital for Sick Children,
Yorkhill, Glasgow G3 8SJ
Stillbirth and Neonatal Death Society
28 Portland Place
London W1N 4DE

New Zealand:

Compassionate Friends New Zealand
9 Welles Street
Ranfurly, Otago

Stillbirth and Neonatal Death Support
30 Church Street
Palmerston North

Bibliography

BOOKS

Ainsworth-Smith, I. *Letting Go.* London: SPCK, 1982.

Ammerman, L.T. (Ed.). *Of Such Is the Kingdom.* Nashville: Abingdon-Cokesbury, 1954.

Aries, P. (Ed.). *Death in America.* Philadelphia: University of Pennsylvania Press, 1975.

Armstrong, O.V. *Comfort for Those Who Mourn.* Nashville: Parthenon Press, 1930.

Arnold, J.H., and P.B. Gemma. *A Child Dies: A Family Portrait.* Rockville, MD: Aspen Systems Corporation, 1983.

Becker, E. *The Denial of Death.* New York: Macmillan, 1973.

Berezin, N. *After a Loss in Pregnancy: Help for Families Affected by Miscarriage, a Stillbirth, or the Loss of a Newborn.* New York: Simon and Schuster, 1982.

Berg, B. *Nothing to Cry About.* New York: Harper & Row, 1981.

Bernstein, J.E. *Loss and How to Cope with It.* New York: Seabury Press, 1977.

Blackburn, L.B. *Timothy Duck.* Omaha, NE: Centering Corporation, 1987.

Borg, S., and J. Lasker. *When Pregnancy Fails: Families Coping with Miscarriage, Stillbirth and Loss of a Newborn.* New York: Bantam Books, 1988.

Bowlby, J. *Attachment and Loss. Vol. 3, Loss.* New York: Basic Books, 1980.

Bozarth-Campbell, A. *Life Is Goodbye, Life Is Hello.* Minneapolis: CompCare Publications, 1982.

Brown, M.W. *The Dead Bird.* New York: Dell Publishing Company, Inc., 1979.

Bush, M. *The Adventure Called Death.* New York: B. Wheelwright Company, 1950.

Church, D. *Facing Death, Finding Love.* Lower Lake, CA: Aslan Publishers, 1994.

Church, M.J., H. Chazin, and F.M. Ewald. *When a Baby Dies.* Oak Brook, IL: The Compassionate Friends, 1981.

Clayton, P.J. Bereavement and Its Management. In *Handbook of Affective Disorders,* E.S. Paykel (Ed.). Edinburgh: Churchill Livingstone.

Cohn, J. *I Had a Friend Named Peter.* New York: William Morrow and Company, Inc., 1987.

Cohn, J. *Molly's Rosebush.* Chicago: Albert Whitman Press.

D'Arcy, P. *Song for Sarah.* Wheaton, IL: Harold Shaw Publishers, 1981.

Davidson, G.W. *Understanding Death of a Wished-For Child.* Springfield, IL: OGR Service Corp, 1979.

————. *Understanding Mourning.* Minneapolis: Augsburg, 1984.

Davis, D.L. *Empty Cradle, Broken Heart.* Golden, CO: Fulcrum Publishing, 1991.

Defrain, J., J. Taylor, and L. Ernst. *Stillborn–The Invisible Death.* Lexington, MA: D.C. Hath/Lexington Books, 1986.

DeHamer, N., and J. Morrow. *Good Mourning: Help and Understanding in Time of Parent Loss.* Waco, TX: Word Publishing, 1989.

Dodd, R.V. *Helping Children Cope with Death.* Scottdale, PA: Herald Press, 1984.

Dodge, N., and J. M. Lamb Sr. *Sharing with Thumpy.* Springfield, IL: Prairie Lark Press, 1985.

_____. *Thumpy's Story.* Springfield, IL: Prairie Lark Press, 1983.

Edelstein, L. *Maternal Bereavement: Coping with the Unexpected Death of a Child.* New York: Praeger, 1984.

Ewing, S. *Newborn Death.* Springfield, IL: Creative Marketing, 1982.

Ewy, D., and R. Ewy. *Death of a Dream.* New York: E.P. Dutton, Inc., 1984.

Fallaci, O. *Letter to a Child Never Born.* New York: Simon and Schuster, 1975.

Feher, L. *The Psychology of Birth.* New York: Continuum, 1981.

Fischhoff, J., and N.O. Brohl. *Before and After My Child Died: A Collection of Parent's Experiences.* Detroit, MI: Emmons-Fairfield Publishing Co., 1981.

Friedman, R., and B. Gradstein. *Surviving Pregnancy Loss.* Boston: Little, Brown and Company, 1982.

Fritsch, J., and S. Ilse. *The Anguish of Loss.* Maple Plain, MN: Wintergreen Press, 1988.

Galinsky, H. *Beginnings.* New York: Houghton Mifflin, 1976.

Garfield, C.A.A. A Child Dies. In *Stress and Survival,* C.A. Garfield (Ed.). St. Louis: C.V. Mosby Co., 1979, pp. 314-317.

Grollman, E.A. (Ed.). *Explaining Death to Children.* Boston: Beacon Press, 1967.

_____. *Talking About Death: A Dialogue Between Parent and Child.* Boston: Beacon Press, 1976.

Gryte, M. *No New Baby.* Omaha, NE: Centering Corp.

Harper, A. *Remembering Michael.* London: The Stillbirth and Neonatal Death Society, 1994.

Harrison, H. *The Premature Baby Book.* New York: St. Martin's Press, 1983.

Hayford, J. *I'll Hold You in Heaven: Healing and Hope for the Parent Who Has Lost a Child Through Miscarriage Stillbirth, Abortion, or Early Infant Death.* Ventura, CA: Regal Press, 1990.

Heegaard, M.E. *Coping with Death and Grief.* Minneapolis: Lerner Publications, 1990.

Hey, V., C. Itzin, L. Saunders, and M. Speakman. *Hidden Loss: Miscarriage and Ectopic Pregnancy.* London: The Women's Press, 1989.

Hollingsworth, C.E., and R.O. Pasnau (Eds.). *The Family in Mourning: Guide for Health Care Professionals.* New York: Grune and Stratton, 1977.

Huntley, T. *Helping Children Grieve.* Minneapolis: Augsburg Press, 1991.

Ilse, S. *Another Baby? Maybe. . . .* Maple Plain, MN: Wintergreen Press, 1996.

_____. *Empty Arms: Coping with Miscarriage, Stillbirth and Infant Death.* Maple Plain, MN: Wintergreen Press, 1990.

_____. *Giving Care–Taking Care.* Maple Plain, MN: Wintergreen Press, 1996.

_____. and L.H. Burns. *Miscarriage: A Shattered Dream.* Maple Plain, MN: Wintergreen Press, 1985.

Jackson, E.N. *Telling a Child About Death.* New York: Channel Press, 1965.

————. *Understanding Grief.* Nashville: Abingdon Press, 1957.

————. *You and Your Grief.* New York: Hawthorn Books, Inc., 1962.

Jewett, C. *Helping Children Cope with Separation and Loss.* Harvard, MA: Harvard Common Press, 1982.

Jensen, A.H. *Healing Grief.* Redmond, Washington: Medic Press, 1980.

Jimenez, S.L.M. *The Other Side of Pregnancy: Coping with Miscarriage and Stillbirth.* Englewood Cliffs, NJ: Prentice-Hall, 1982.

Johnson, J., and M. Johnson. *Newborn Death.* Grand Neck, NY: Centering Corporation, 1982.

————. *Tell Me Papa.* Grand Neck, NY: Centering Corporation, 1978.

————. *Where's Jess?* Omaha, NB: Centering Corporation, 1982.

Klaus, M., and J.H. Kennell. *Maternal-Infant Bonding.* St. Louis: C.V. Mosby Company, 1976.

————. *Parent-Infant Bonding.* St. Louis: C.V. Mosby, 1982.

————. *The Beginnings of Parent-Infant Attachment.* New York: New American Library, 1983.

————. Caring for Parents of Stillborn or an Infant Who Dies. In *Maternal-Infant Bonding,* J.H. Klaus and M.H. Kennell (Eds.). St. Louis: The C.V. Mosby Company, 1982, pp. 209-239.

Knapp, R.J. *Beyond Endurance: When a Child Dies.* New York: Schocken Books, 1986.

Kohn, I., and P. Moffitt. *Silent Sorrow: Pregnancy Loss Guidance and Support for You and Your Family.* New York, NY: Delacorte Press/Bantam Doubleday Dell Publishing Group, Inc., 1992.

Kohner, N., and A. Henley. *When a Baby Dies.* San Francisco: Harper Collins Publishers, 1995.

————. *Miscarriage, Stillbirth and Neonatal Death: Guidelines for Professionals.* London, 1991.

Kohner, N. *A Dignified Ending: Recommendation for Good Practice in the Disposal of Bodies and Remains of Babies Born Dead Before the Legal Age of Viability.* London: The Stillbirth and Neonatal Death Society, 1992.

Kolf, J.C. *When Will I Stop Hurting: Dealing with a Recent Death.* Grand Rapids, MI: Baker Book House, 1987.

Kotzwinkle, W. *Swimmer in the Secret Sea.* New York: Avon, 1975.

Kübler-Ross, E. *Death–The Final Stage of Growth.* Englewood Cliffs, NJ: Prentice-Hall, 1975.

Kübler-Ross, E. *On Children and Death.* New York: Macmillan Publishing Co., 1983

Lamb, Sr. J.M. (Ed.). *Bittersweet . . . Hello Goodbye: A Resource in Planning Farewell Rituals When a Baby Dies.* Springfield, IL: Prairie Lark Press, 1988.

Landorf, J. *Mourning Song.* Old Tappan, NJ: Fleming H. Revell Co., 1974.

Langone, J. *Death Is a Noun.* Boston: Little, Brown, and Company, 1972.

Leon, I.G. *When a Baby Dies: Psychotherapy for Pregnancy and Newborn Loss.* New Haven, CN: Yale University Press, 1990.

Limbo, R.K., and S.R. Wheeler. *When a Baby Dies: Handbook for Healing and Helping.* LaCrosse, Wisconsin: Resolve Through Sharing, 1986.

Lister, M., and S. Lovell. *Healing Together–For Couples Whose Baby Dies.* Omaha, NE: Centering Corp., 1991.

MacFarlane, J.A., D.M. Smith, and D.H. Garrow. *The Relationship Between Mother and Neonate in the Place of Birth,* S. Kitzinger and J.A. Davis (Eds.). New York: Oxford University Press, 1978.

Mander, R. *Loss and Bereavement in Childbearing.* Oxford: Blackwell Scientific Publications, 1994.

Manning, D. *Comforting Those Who Grieve: A Guide for Helping Others.* San Francisco: Harper and Row, 1985.

————. *Don't Take My Grief Away from Me.* San Francisco: Harper and Row for Insight Books, 1984.

Massanari, J., and A. Massanari. *Our Life with Caleb.* Philadelphia: Fortress Press, 1976.

Mellonie, B., and R. Ingpen. *Lifetimes.* New York: Bantam Books Inc., 1983.

Miles, M. *The Grief of Parents When a Child Dies.* Oak Brook, IL: The Compassionate Friends, Inc. 1978.

Mitscherlich, A., and M. Mitscherlich. *The Inability to Mourn.* New York: Grove Press, 1975.

Moulder, C. *Miscarriage: Women's Experiences and Needs.* London: Pandora, 1990.

Oehler, J. *The Frog Family's Baby Dies.* (coloring book) Durham, NC: Duke University Medical Center, 1978.

Osgood, J. (Ed.). *Meditations for Bereaved Parents.* Sunriver, OR: Gilgal Publications, 1983.

Osterweis, M., F. Solomon, and M. Green (Eds.). Bereavement: Reactions, Consequences, and Care (Report by the Committee for the Study of Health Consequences of the Stress of Bereavement, Institute of Medicine, National Academy of Sciences). Washington, DC: National Academy Press, 1984.

Palinski, C.O., and H. Pizer. *Coping with a Miscarriage.* New York: New American Library, 1980.

Panuthos, C., and C. Romeo. *Ended Beginnings: Healing Childbearing Losses.* South Hadley, MA: Begin & Garvey Pub. Co. Inc., 1984.

Papenbrock, P. L., and R.F. Voss, F. *Children's Grief.* Redmond, WA: Medic Publishing Company, 1988.

Parkes, C.M., and R.S. Weiss. *Recovery from Bereavement.* New York: Basic Books, Inc., 1983.

Parrott, C. *Parents' Grief.* Redmond, WA: Medic Publishing Company, 1992.

Peppers, L.G., and R.J. Knapp. *How to Go on Living After the Death of a Baby.* Atlanta: Peachtree Publishers, 1985.

————. *Motherhood and Mourning.* New York: Praeger Publishers, 1980.

Pizer, H., and C. Palinski. *Coping with Miscarriage.* New York: American Library/Plumbe Books, 1980.

Rando, T.A. *Grief, Dying and Death.* Champaign, IL: Research Press Co., 1984.

————. *Grieving: How to Go on Living When Someone You Love Dies.* Lexington, MA: C.Heath/Lexington Books, 1988.

————. *Parental Loss of a Child.* Champaign, IL: Research Press Company, 1986.

Richter, E. *Losing Someone You Love.* New York: G. P. Putnam's Sons, 1986.

Rosenblatt, P.C. *Bitter, Bitter Tears.* Minneapolis: University of Minnesota Press, 1983.

Rudolph, M. *Should the Children Know?* New York: Schocken Books, 1978.

Sahler, O.J.Z. *The Child and Death.* St. Louis: C.V. Mosby Company, 1978.

Sanford, D. *It Must Hurt a Lot.* Portland, OR: Multnomah Press, 1986.

Savage, J.A. *Mourning Unlived Lives.* Wilmette, IL: Chiron Publications, 1989.

Schaefer, D., and C. Lyons. *How Do We Tell the Children?* New York: Newmarket Press, 1986.

Schatz, W. *Healing a Father's Grief.* Redmond, WA: Medic Publishing Company, 1984.

Scherago, M. *Sibling Grief.* Redmond, WA: Medic Publishing Company, 1987.

Schiff, H.S. *The Bereaved Parent.* New York: Penguin Books, 1978.

————. *Living Through Mourning.* New York: Penguin Books, 1987.

Schinn, M. *Biography of a Baby.* Boston: Houghton Mifflin Company, 1900.

Schowalter, J. *Children and Death: Perspectives from Birth to Adolescence.* New York: Praeger & Co., 1987.

Schuchardt, E. *Why Is This Happening to Me?* Minneapolis: Augsburg, 1989.

Schwab, J.J., J.M. Chalmers, S.J. Conroy, P.B. Farris, and R.E. Markush. Studies in Grief: A Preliminary Report. In *Bereavement: Its Psychosocial Aspects,* B. Schoenberg, I. Gerber, A. Wiener, A.I. Kutscher, D. Peretz, and A.C. Carr (Eds.). New York: Columbia University Press, 1975.

Schweibert, P., and P. Kirk. *When Hello Means Goodbye.* Portland, OR: Perinatal Loss, 1985.

Sims, A. *Am I Still a Sister?* Albuquerque, NM: Big A and Company, 1986.

Slater, P. *Children in the New England Mind: In Death and in Life.* Hamden, CT: Archer Books, 1977.

Smith, D.B. *A Taste of Blackberries.* New York: Harper & Row Publishers, 1973.

Stein, S.B. *About Dying.* New York: Walker and Company, 1974.

Stinson, R., and P. Stinson. *The Long Dying of Baby Andrew.* Boston: Little, Brown, and Company, 1983.

Tengbom, M. *Help for Bereaved Parents.* St. Louis: Concordia Publishing House, 1981.

Varley, S. *Badger's Parting Gifts.* New York: Lothrop, Lee and Shepard Books, 1984.

Viorst, J. *The Tenth Good Thing about Barney.* New York: Atheneum Publishers, 1971.

Vogel, L.J. *Helping a Child Understand Death.* Philadelphia: Fortress Press, 1975.

Vredevelt, P.W. *Empty Arms: Emotional Support for Those Who Have Suffered Miscarriage or Stillbirth.* Portland, OR: Multnomah Press, 1984.

Westberg, G.E. *Good Grief.* Philadelphia: Fortress Press, 1971.

Westphal, M. *God, Guilt, and Death.* Bloomington: Indiana University Press, 1984.
Wiesbe, D.W. *Gone but Not Lost: Grieving the Death of a Child.* Grand Rapids, MI: Baker Book House, 1991.
Wilcox, S., and M. Sutton. *Understanding Death and Dying: An Interdisciplinary Approach.* Sherman Oaks, CA: Alfred Publishing Company, 1981.
Wolfelt, A. *Helping Children Cope with Grief.* Muncie, IN: Accelerated Development Inc., 1983.
Wolterstorff, N. *Lament for a Son.* Grand Rapids, MI: Eerdmans, 1987.
Woods, J.R., and J.L. Esposito (Eds.). *Pregnancy Loss: Medical Therapeutics and Practical Considerations.* Baltimore: William and Wilkins, 1987.

PERIODICALS

Baran, A., R. Pannor, and A. Sorosky. "The Lingering Pain of Surrendering a Child." *Psychology Today,* June, 1977.
Barry, H.J. Jr. "Significance of Maternal Bereavement Before the Age Eight in Psychiatric Patients." *Archives of Neurological Psychiatry,* 62, (1949): 630-637.
Beard, R.W., J. Beckley, D. Black, C. Brewer, Y. Craig, A. Hill, H. Jolly, E. Lewis, H. Lewis, and S. Limerick. "Help for Parents After Stillbirth." *British Medical Journal,* 1, (1978): 172-173.
Beck, M., I. Wickelgren, V. Quade, and P. Wingert. "Miscarriages." *Newsweek,* August 15, 1988: 46-52.
Benfield, D.G., S.A. Leib, and J.H. Vollman. "Grief Response of Parents to Neonatal Death and Parent Participation in Deciding Care." *Pediatrics,* 62(2), (1978): 171-177.
Bergman, A. "Psychological Aspects of Sudden Unexpected Death in Infants and Children." *Pediatric Clinics of North America,* 21, (February, 1974): 115-121.
Bibring, G. "Some Considerations of the Psychological Processes in Pregnancy." *Psychoanalytic Study of Children,* 14, (1959): 810-812.
Boue, J., A. Boue, P. Lazar, and I. Gueguen. "Outcome of Pregnancies Following a Spontaneous Abortion with Chromosomal Anomalies." *American Journal of Obstetrics and Gynecology,* 116(6), (July, 1973): 806-811.
Breuer, J. "Sharing a Tragedy." *American Journal of Nursing,* 76, (1976): 758-759.
Bruce, S. "Reactions of Nurses and Mothers to Stillborns." *Nursing Outlook,* 10, (1962): 88ff.
Cain, A., and B. Cain. "On Replacing a Child." *American Academy of Child Psychiatry,* 3, (1964): 443-455.
Carr, D., and S.F. Knupp. "Grief and Perinatal Loss: A Community Approach to Support." *Journal of Obstetric, Gynecologic, and Neonatal Nursing,* 14, (1985): 130-139.
Chance, G.W., M. Beaudry, M. MacMurray, M. Pendray, and D. Shea. "Support for Parents Experiencing Perinatal Loss." *Canadian Medical Association Journal* 129(4), (1983): 335-339.

Chez, R. "Helping Patients and Doctors Cope with Perinatal Death." *Contemporary OB/GYN*, 20, (1982): 98.

Coffin, W.S. Jr. "My Son Beat Me to the Grave." *The Lutheran Standard,* (April 20, 1984): 4-7.

Cohen, L., Z. Zilkha, J. Middleton, and N. O'Donnohue. "Perinatal Mortality: Assisting Parental Affirmation." *American Journal of Orthopsychiatry* 48(4)4, (1978): 727-731.

Condon, J.T. "Management of Established Pathological Grief Reaction After Stillbirth." *American Journal of Psychiatry*, 143, (1986): 987-992.

Condon, J.T. "Prevention of Emotional Disability Following Stillbirth–The Role of the Obstetric Team" *Australian and New Zealand Journal of Obstetrics and Gynecology*, 27(4), (1987): 323-329.

Courtney, S.E., N. Thomas, and B.K. Predmore. "Reverse Transport of the Deceased Neonate–An aid to Mourning." *American Journal of Perinatalogy*, 2(3), (1985): 217-220.

Crout, T.K. "Caring for the Mother of a Stillborn Baby." *Nursing '80,* 10, (1980): 70-73.

Davidson, G.W. "Death of the Wished-For Child: A Case Study." *Death Education*, 1, (1977): 265-277.

Davis, D.L., M. Stewart, and R.J. Harmon. "Perinatal Loss: Providing Emotional Support for Bereaved Parents." *Birth*, 15(4), (1988): 242-246.

Davis, J.A. "Management of Perinatal Loss of a Twin." *British Medical Journal*, 297(6663), (1988): 1613.

Dyregrov, A., and S.B. Matthiesen. "Anxiety and Vulnerability in Parents Following the Death of an Infant." *Scandinavian Journal of Psychology*, 28(1), (1987): 16-25.

————. "Similarities and Differences in Mother's and Father's Grief Following the Death of an Infant." *Scandinavian Journal of Psychology*, 28(1), (1987): 1-15.

Eliot, T.D. "Of the Shadow of Death." *Annals of the American Academy of Political and Social Science*, 229, (1943): 87-99.

Elliot, B.A. "Neonatal Death: Reflections for Parents." *Pediatrics*, 62(1), (1978): 100-102.

Elliot, B.A. and H.A. Hein. "Neonatal Death: Reflections for Physicians." *Pediatrics*, 62(1), (1978): 96-99.

Fickling, K.F. "Stillborn Studies: Ministering to Bereaved Parents." *The Journal of Pastoral Care*, 47(3), (1993): 217-227.

Furlong, R.M., and J.C. Hobbins. "Grief in the Perinatal Period." *Obstetrics and Gynecology*, 61(4), (1983): 497-500.

Furman, E.P. "The Death of a Newborn: Care of Parents." *Birth Family Journal*, 5, (1978): 214-218.

Giles, P.F.H. "Reactions of Women to Perinatal Death." *Australia/New Zealand Journal of Obstetrics and Gynecology*, 10, (1970): 207-210.

Gilson, G. "Care of the Family Who Has Lost a Newborn." *Post Graduate Medicine*, 60, (December, 1976): 67-70.

Hagan, J.M. "Infant Death–Nursing Interaction and Intervention with Grieving Families." *Nursing Forum*, 13, (1974): 373-385.

Harmon, R.J., A.D. Glicken, and R.E. Siegel. "Neonatal Loss in the Intensive Care Nursery: Effects on Maternal Grieving and a Program for Intervention" *Journal of the American Academy of Child Psychiatry*, (1984): 68-71.

Helmrath, T.A., and Steinitz, E.M. "Death of an Infant: Parental Grieving and the Failure of Social Support." *The Journal of Family Practice*, 6(4), (1978): 785-790.

Hildebrand, W.L., and R.L. Schreiner. "Helping Parents Cope with Perinatal Death." *American Family Physician*, 22(5), (1980): 121-125.

Jackson, P.L. "When the Baby Isn't Perfect." *American Journal of Nursing*, 85(4), (1985): 396-399.

Jensen, J., and R. Zahourek. "Depression in Mothers Who Have Lost a Newborn." *Rocky Mountain Medical Journal*, 69, (1972): 61-63.

Johnson, J. "Guiding Children Through Grief." *Mothering*, 51, (1989): 29-35.

Johnson, J. "When Things Go Wrong: What to Do If Your Newborn Dies." *Mothering*, 39, (1986): 26-29.

Kennel, J.H., H. Slyter, and M. Klaus. "The Mourning Response of Parents to the Death of a Newborn." *New England Journal of Medicine*, 283 (1970): 344-349.

Kirkley-Best, E., and K.R. Kellner. "The Forgotten Grief: A Review of the Psychology of Stillbirth." *American Journal of Orthopsychiatry*, 52, (1982): 420-429.

Kirkley-Best, E., and C. VanDevere. "The Hidden Family Grief: An Overview of Grief in the Family Following Perinatal Death." *International Journal of Family Psychiatry*, 7(4), (1986): 419-437.

Koch, J. "When Children Meet Death." *Psychology Today*, (November 1977): 64-66.

Kowalski, K. "Managing Perinatal Loss." *Clinical OB/GYN*, 23, (1980): 1113-1123.

Kowalski, K., and W. Bowes. "Parents' Response to a Stillborn Baby." *Contemporary OB/GYN*, 6, (1976): 53-57.

Krell, R. and L. Rabkin. "The Effects of Sibling Death on the Surviving Child: A Family Perspective." *Family Process*, 18, (1970): 471-477.

LaFerla, J.J., and R.S. Good. "Helping Patients Cope with Pregnancy Loss." *Contemporary OB/GYN*, 25(4), (1985): 14-19.

LaRoche, C., M. Lalinec-Michaud, F. Engelsmann, N. Fuller, M. Copp, L. McQuade-Soldatos, and R. Azima. "Grief Reactions to Perinatal Death: A Follow-Up Study." *Canadian Journal of Psychiatry*, 29, (1984): 14-19.

Lauritsen, J.G. "Genetic Aspects of Spontaneous Abortions." *Danish Medical Bulletin*, 24(5), (October, 1977): 169-188.

Leon, I.G. "Psychodynamics of Perinatal Loss." *Psychiatry*, 49, (1986): 312-324.

Leppert, P.C., and B.S. Pahlka. "Grieving Characteristics After Spontaneous Abortion: A Management Approach." *Obstetrics and Gynecology*, 64(1), (1984): 119-122.

Lewis, E. "(The) Management of Stillbirth: Coping with an Unreality." *Lancet*, 2, 1976: 610-620.

_____. "Mourning by the Family After a Stillbirth or Neonatal Death." *Archives of Disease in Childhood*, 54, (1979): 303-306.

Lewis, E., and A. Page. "Failure to Mourn a Stillbirth: An Overlooked Catastrophe." *British Journal of Medical Psychology*, 51, (1978): 237-241.

Limbo, R.K., and S.R. Wheeler. "Coping with Unexpected Outcomes. *NAACOG Update Series*, 5(3), (1986): 1-8.

_____. "Family-Centered Care for Bereaved Families" *The Cybele Report*, 6(3), (1985): 3-6.

Lindermann, E. "Symptomatology and Management of Acute Grief." *American Journal of Psychiatry*, 101(2), (1944): 141-148.

Mandell, F., M. McLain, and R. Reece. "The Sudden Infant Death Syndrome: Siblings and Their Place in the Family." *Annals of the New York Academy of Sciences*, 533, (1988): 129-131.

Martocchio, B.C. "Grief and Bereavement: Healing Through Hurt." *Nursing Clinics of North America*, 2, (1985): 327-341.

Mills, G. C. "Books to Help Children Understand Death." *American Journal of Nursing*, 79, (1979): 291-295.

Moriarity, D. "The Right to Mourn." *MS Magazine*, (November, 1982): 79-80.

Murray, J., and V.J. Callan. "Predicting Adjustment to Perinatal Death." *British Journal of Medical Psychology*, 61(3), (1988): 237-244.

Nichol, M.T., J. Tompkins, N. Campbell, and G. Syme. "Maternal Grieving Response After Perinatal Death." *Medical Journal of Australia*, 144, (1986): 287-289.

O'Connor, K. "How to Talk to Your Child About Death." *Liguorian*, 68, (1980): 34-38.

Parkes, C.M. "The First Year of Bereavement." *Psychiatry*, 33, (1970): 444-467.

Peppers, L.G., and R.J. Knapp. "Maternal Reactions to Involuntary Fetal/Infant Death." *Psychiatry*, 43, (1980): 155-159.

Phillips, S.G. "Coping with Miscarriage . . . My Own Experience." *American Baby*, (July 1980): 38-39.

Phipps, S. "The Subsequent Pregnancy After Stillbirth: Anticipatory Parenthood in the Face of Uncertainty." *International Journal of Psychiatry and Medicine*, 15, (1985): 243-264.

Pizer, H., and Palinski, C. "Coping with a Miscarriage." *American Baby*, (September 1981): 42ff.

Pozanski, E.O. "The Replacement Child: A Saga of Unresolved Parental Grief." *Behavioral Pediatrics*, 81(6), (1972): 1190-1193.

Putnam, C.H. "Losing Jacob." *The Sunday Camera Magazine* (Boulder, Colorado), (November 19, 1989): 1-9.

Queenan, J. "Never Underestimate the Help You Can Offer Bereaved Parents." *Contemporary Obstetrics and Gynecology,* 12, (1978): 9-10.

Rosenblatt, P.G., and L.H. Burns. "Long-Term Effects of Perinatal Loss." *Journal of Family Issues,* 7(3), (1986): 237-253.

Rowe, J., R. Clyman, C. Green, C. Mikkelsen, J. Haight, and L. Ataide. "Follow-Up of Families Who Experience Perinatal Death." *Pediatrics,* 62(2), (1978): 166-170.

Rubin, S.S. "Mourning Distinct from Melancholia: The Resolution of Bereavement." *British Journal of Medical Psychology,* 57, (1984): 339-345.

Saylor, D.E. "Nursing Response to Mothers of Stillborn Infants." *Journal of Obstetrical and Gynecological Nursing,* 6(4), (1977): 39-42.

Schodt, C. "Grief in Adolescent Mothers After an Infant Death." *Image,* (1982): 20-25.

Scrimshaw, S.C.M., and D.M.S. March. "I Had a Baby Sister but She Only Lasted One Day." *Journal of the American Medical Association,* 251(6), (Feb. 10, 1984): 732-733.

Sculpholme, A. "Coping with the Unexpected Outcomes of Pregnancy." *Journal of Obstetrical and Gynecological Nursing,* 7(3), (1978): 36-39.

Seitz, P.M., and L.H. Warrick. "Perinatal Death: The Grieving Mother." *American Journal of Nursing,* 74(11), (1974): 2028-2033.

Speck, W.T., and J.H. Kennell. "Management of Perinatal Death." *Pediatrics in Review,* 2, (1980): 59-62.

Sperhac, A.M. "Sudden Infant Death Syndrome." *Nurse Practitioner,* 7(8), (1982): 38-44.

Stack, J.M. "The Psychodynamics of Spontaneous Abortion." *The American Journal of Orthopsychiatry,* 54(1), (1984): 162-167.

Stack, J.M. "Spontaneous Abortion and Grieving." *American Family Physician,* 21(5), (1980): 99-102.

Stephany, T. "Early Miscarriage: Are We too Quick to Dismiss the Pain?" *RN,* 45, (1982): 89.

Stierman, E.D. "Emotional Aspects of Perinatal Death." *Clinical Obstetrics and Gynecology,* 30(2), (1987): 352-361.

Stringham, J.G., J.H. Riley, and A. Ross. "Silent Birth: Mourning a Stillborn Baby." *Social Work,* 27(4), (1982): 322-327.

Swanson-Kauffman, K.M. "Caring in the Instance of Unexpected Early Miscarriage." *Topics in Clinical Nursing,* 8(2), (1986): 37-46.

Theut, S.K., F. Pedersen, M. Zaslow, R. Gain, B. Rabinovich, and J. Morihisa. "Perinatal Loss and Parental Bereavement." *American Journal of Psychiatry,* 146(5), (1989): 635-639.

Tizard. J.P.M. "Mourning Made Easier if Parents Can View Body of Neonate." *OB/Gyn News,* 11(21), (1976): 35.

Tomsyck, R.R. "The Grief of a Mother/Physician on the Death of Her Infant." *Journal of American Medical Women's Association,* 43(2), (1988): 51-57.

Tudehope, D.I., J. Iredell, D. Rodgers, and A. Gunn. "Neonatal Death: Grieving Families." *Medical Journal of Australia,* 144, (1986): 290-292.

Videka-Sherman, L., and M. Lieberman. "The Effects of Self-Help and Psychotherapy Intervention on Child Loss: The Limits of Recovery." *American Journal of Orthopsychiatry*, 55(1), (1985): 70-82.

Wall-Hass, C.L. "Women's Perceptions of First Trimester Spontaneous Abortion." *Journal of Obstetric, Gynecologic, and Neonatal Nursing*, 8(1), (1985): 50-53.

Wasserman, A.L. "Helping Families Get Through the Holidays After the Death of a Child." *American Journal of Diseases of Children*, 142(12), (1988): 1284-1286.

Wetzal, S.K. "Are We Ignoring the Needs of the Woman with a Spontaneous Abortion?" *American Journal of Maternal Child Nursing*, 7, (1982): 258-259.

Wilson, A.L., L. Fenton, D. Stevens, and D. Soule. "The Death of a Newborn Twin: An Analysis of Parental Bereavement." *Pediatrics*, 70, (1982): 587-591.

Wilson, A.L., D. Witzke, L. Fenton, D. Soule. "Parental Response to Perinatal Death: Mother-Father Differences." *American Journal of Diseases of Children*, 139(12), (1986): 1235-1238.

Wilson, A.L., and D.J. Soule. "The Role of a Self-Help Group in Working with Parents of a Stillborn Baby." *Death Education*, 5, (1981): 175-186.

Wolff, J., P. Nielson, and P. Schiller. "The Emotional Reaction to Stillbirth." *American Journal of Obstetrics and Gynecology*, 108, (1970): 73-77.

Wong, D.L. "Bereavement: The Empty Mother Syndrome." *American Journal of Maternal Child Nursing*, 5, (1980): 384-389.

Woodward, S., A. Pope, W. Robson, and O. Hagan. "Bereavement Counseling After Sudden Infant Death." *British Medical Journal*, 290, (1985): 363-365.

Wortman, C.B., and R.C. Silver. "The Myths of Coping with Loss." *Journal of Consulting and Clinical Psychiatry*, 57(3), (1989): 349-357.

York, C., and J. Stichler. "Cultural Grief Expressions Following Infant Death." *Dimensions of Critical Care Nursing*, 4(2), (1985): 120-127.

Zahourek, R., and J.S. Jensen. "Grieving and the Loss of a Newborn." *American Journal of Nursing*, 73(5), (1973): 836-839.

Zeanah, C.H. "Adaptation Following Perinatal Loss: A Critical Review." *Journal of the American Academy of Child and Adolescent Psychiatry*, 28(3), (1988): 467-480.

THESIS RESEARCH

Davis, D.L. "Perinatal Loss: The Mother's Experience with Grief, Resolution and Subsequent Child." PhD dissertation, Department of Psychology, University of Massachusetts, Amherst, 1986.

Dixon, R. "Funeral and the Grieving Process." DMin thesis, University of Dubuque Library, Dubuque, IA, 1983.

Kowalski, K. "Perinatal Death: An Ethnomethodological Study of Factors Influencing Parental Bereavement." PhD dissertation, Department of Sociology, University of Colorado, Boulder, 1984.

Merrill, S. "Miscarriage: Fathers and Social Support." Master's thesis, University of Wisconsin, Eau Claire, 1986.

Moe, T. "Ministry to Families Suffering from Miscarriage, Stillbirth, and Neonatal Loss." DMin thesis, Bethel Seminary, St. Paul, MN, 1993.

Wales, A.H. "Ministering to Ministers: Death in the Manse." DMin thesis, University of Dubuque Library, Dubuque, IA, 1991.

Index

Page numbers followed by the letter "t" indicate tables.

Order Your Own Copy of
This Important Book for Your Personal Library!

PASTORAL CARE IN PREGNANCY LOSS
A Ministry Long Needed

_____in hardbound at $39.95 (ISBN: 0-7890-0124-1)

_____in softbound at $19.95 (ISBN: 0-7890-0196-9)

COST OF BOOKS_____

OUTSIDE USA/CANADA/
MEXICO: ADD 20%_____

POSTAGE & HANDLING_____
*(US: $3.00 for first book & $1.25
for each additional book)
Outside US: $4.75 for first book
& $1.75 for each additional book)*

SUBTOTAL_____

IN CANADA: ADD 7% GST_____

STATE TAX_____
*(NY, OH & MN residents, please
add appropriate local sales tax)*

FINAL TOTAL_____
*(If paying in Canadian funds,
convert using the current
exchange rate. UNESCO
coupons welcome.)*

☐ **BILL ME LATER:** ($5 service charge will be added)
(Bill-me option is good on US/Canada/Mexico orders only;
not good to jobbers, wholesalers, or subscription agencies.)

☐ Check here if billing address is different from
shipping address and attach purchase order and
billing address information.

Signature_____

☐ **PAYMENT ENCLOSED: $**_____

☐ **PLEASE CHARGE TO MY CREDIT CARD.**

☐ Visa   ☐ MasterCard   ☐ AmEx   ☐ Discover

Account # _____

Exp. Date _____

Signature _____

Prices in US dollars and subject to change without notice.

NAME _____

INSTITUTION _____

ADDRESS _____

CITY _____

STATE/ZIP _____

COUNTRY _____ COUNTY (NY residents only) _____

TEL _____ FAX _____

E-MAIL_____
May we use your e-mail address for confirmations and other types of information? ☐ Yes   ☐ No

Order From Your Local Bookstore or Directly From
The Haworth Press, Inc.
10 Alice Street, Binghamton, New York 13904-1580 • USA
TELEPHONE: 1-800-HAWORTH (1-800-429-6784) / Outside US/Canada: (607) 722-5857
FAX: 1-800-895-0582 / Outside US/Canada: (607) 772-6362
E-mail: getinfo@haworth.com
PLEASE PHOTOCOPY THIS FORM FOR YOUR PERSONAL USE.

BOF96

MORE TITLES OF RELATED INTEREST FROM THE HAWORTH PRESS, INC.

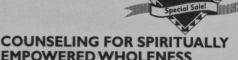

THEOLOGICAL CONTEXT FOR PASTORAL CAREGIVING

Word in Deed

The Rev. Howard W. Stone, PhD

NEW!

"THIS BOOK WILL HELP THE PLANT OF PASTORAL CARE TO FLOURISH AND FLOWER IN THE CHALLENGING YEARS JUST AHEAD."
—Howard Clinebell, PhD, Author, *Ecotherapy: Healing Ourselves, Healing the Earth*

In **Theological Context for Pastoral Caregiving**, Howard W. Stone helps his fellow pastors and worship leaders provide effective and faithful pastoral care and counseling through the study of the correlation between pastoral care and theology. You will learn that in order for pastoral care to be faithful it must have a theological base to shape the caregiving experience. At the same time, theology must be informed by the needs and experiences of the people being served and by the ministry of pastoral care. By relating these two issues, you gain a unique viewpoint not offered by books with simply a psychological focus.

Contents
The Distinctiveness of Pastoral Care • Theological Assessment • The Word • Correlating Theology and Ministry • Spiritual Direction • The Priesthood of All Believers • Acceptance of Self and Spirit • Suffering • Love of God and Neighbor • Pastoral Care as Community Endeavor • Index

$29.95 hard. ISBN: 0-7890-0072-5.
(Outside US/Canada/Mexico: $36.00)
$19.95 soft. ISBN: 0-7890-0125-X.
(Outside US/Canada/Mexico: $24.00)
1996. Available now.174 pp. with Index.

COUNSELING FOR SPIRITUALLY EMPOWERED WHOLENESS

A Hope-Centered Approach

Howard Clinebell, PhD

"CLINEBELL OFFERS IDEAS AND METHODS THAT HELP PLUMB THE DEPTHS OF THE HUMAN SOUL WITH THOSE WHO COME TO US FOR CARE AND COUNSEL."
—Kathleen J. Greider, Assistant Professor of Pastoral Care and Counseling, School of Theology at Claremont

Encourages readers to apply the principles and methods in the book to their own growth and to develop their own growth-centered approaches—approaches that reflect their particular styles and personalities—to counseling, therapy, and education.

Selected Contents
The Goals of Wholeness or Growth Counseling • The Working Principles of Wholeness Counseling • The Flow and Methods of Wholeness Counseling • Spiritual Growth—The Key to All Wholeness • Biblical and Theological Resources for Wholeness Counseling • Wholeness Counseling Through the Stages of Life • Summary and Conclusion: Developing Your Own Wholeness-Centered Approaches to Counseling and Therapy, Education, and Life Enhancement • Notes • Bibliography: For Further Exploration of Growth Counseling • Index • *more*

$39.95 hard. ISBN: 1-56024-902-1.
(Outside US/Canada/Mexico: $48.00)
$14.95 soft. ISBN: 1-56024-903-X.
(Outside US/Canada/Mexico: $18.00)
1995. pp. with Index.

DEALING WITH DEPRESSION

Five Pastoral Interventions
Richard Dayringer, ThD

"The author and his contributors are pointed in their observations that good intentions and basic care are not enough for pastors to help depressed persons. "
—Glen W. Davidson, MDiv, PhD, The Doane Professor and Vice President for Academic Affairs, Doane College; Adjunct Professor of Preventive and Societal Medicine, University of Nebraska Medical Center

$39.95 hard. ISBN: 1-56024-933-1.
(Outside US/Canada/Mexico: $48.00)
$14.95 soft. ISBN: 1-56024-967-6.
(Outside US/Canada/Mexico: $18.00)
1995. 175 pp. with Index.

Explores strategies to enable clergy to identify and help individuals suffering from depression.

Contents
Recognizing Those Who Are Depressed • Transactional Analysis Dealing With Depression • Pastoral Counseling Dealing With Depression • Gestalt Therapy Dealing With Depression • Behavior Therapy in Dealing With Depression • Cognitive Therapy Dealing With Depression • Medical-Religious Case Conference • Clergy Dealing With Depression • Appendixes • Index

Textbooks are available for classroom adoption consideration on a 60–day examination basis. You will receive an invoice payable within 60 days along with the book. **If you decide to adopt the book, your invoice will be cancelled.** Please write to us on your institutional letterhead, indicating the textbook you would like to examine as well as the following information: course title, current text, enrollment, and decision date.

The Haworth Pastoral Press
An imprint of The Haworth Press, Inc.
10 Alice Street, Binghamton,
New York 13904–1580 USA

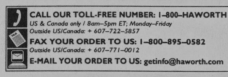